Ethics in the Nuclear Age

Ethics in the Nuclear Age

Strategy, Religious Studies, and the Churches

Edited by
TODD WHITMORE

Southern Methodist University Press
Dallas

First edition, 1989

Requests for permission to reproduce material from this work should be sent to:
    Permissions
    Southern Methodist University Press
    Box 415
    Dallas, Texas 75275

LIBRARY OF CONGRESS CATALOGING-IN-PUBLICATION DATA

Ethics in the nuclear age.
    "This collection of essays is the outgrowth of a two-year workshop
seminar, the Colloquium on Religion and World Affairs, held at the
Divinity School at the University of Chicago"—Pref.
    Bibliography: p.
    Includes index.
    1. Nuclear warfare—Moral and ethical aspects. 2. Nuclear warfare—
Religious aspects—Christianity. 3. Deterrence (Strategy)—Moral and
ethical aspects. 4. Deterrence (Strategy)—Religious aspects—
Christianity. I. Whitmore, Todd, 1957–
U263.E84   1989   172′.42   88-30568
ISBN 0-87074-283-3
ISBN 0-87074-260-4 (pbk.)

The editor and publisher of the present collection wish to extend their gratitude for the permission to reprint two of the essays. David Hollenbach's "Ethics in Distress: Can There Be Just Wars
in the Nuclear Age?" was first published in *The Nuclear Dilemma and the Just War Tradition*,
edited by William V. O'Brien and John Langan, S.J. (Lexington, Mass.: Lexington Books, 1986).
Richard B. Miller's "The Morality of Nuclear Deterrence: Obstacles on the Road to Coherence"
originally appeared in *Horizons* 15, no. 1 (Spring 1988).

For Paul Ramsey   (1913–1988)

Contents

Preface   ix

Introduction   1

I • STRATEGY

1   Ethics and Strategy: The Views of Selected Strategists   13
J. BRYAN HEHIR

II • RELIGIOUS STUDIES

The Problematic of Deterrence

2   The Morality of Nuclear Deterrence: Obstacles on the
Road to Coherence   35
RICHARD B. MILLER

3   Ethics in Distress: Can There Be Just Wars in the
Nuclear Age?   59
DAVID HOLLENBACH, S.J.

4   Bluff or Revenge: The Watershed in
Democratic Deterrence Awareness   79
JOHN HOWARD YODER

The Limits and Possibilities of the New Technologies

5   Deterrence, Defense, or War-Fighting? A Just-War
Analysis of Some Recent Strategic Developments   95
JAMES TURNER JOHNSON

The Discussion in West Germany

6   Problems of Method and Moral Theory in the U.S.
and German Catholic Pastoral Letters on Peace:
A Comparative Explanation   121
JOHN LANGAN, S.J.

7   Nuclear Weapons and Peace: Political Challenge and
     Theological Controversy in West German Protestantism   139
     TRUTZ RENDTORFF

III • THE CHURCHES

8   Peacemaking as an Ethical Category: The Convergence
     of Pacifism and Just War   161
     DUANE K. FRIESEN

9   Reason and Authority in Church Social Documents:
     The Case for Plausibility and Coherence   181
     TODD WHITMORE

     Notes on the Contributors   233
     Index   235

Preface

This collection of essays is the outgrowth of a two-year workshop seminar, the Colloquium on Religion and World Affairs, held at the Divinity School at the University of Chicago. The aim of the seminar was to create a forum that would encourage the further development of the conversation between strategists and the churches which was generated by the 1983 pastoral letter, *The Challenge of Peace*. To this end, the Colloquium sought to enlist the talents and energies of persons in religious studies whose projects address the problem of ethics and strategy in the nuclear age. The sessions were discussions of working papers. Our intention was to facilitate the kind of exchange necessary to respond to the problem of the possession and possible use of nuclear weapons.

To successfully carry off an effort such as this requires the contributions of many persons and institutions. James M. Gustafson, Russell Hardin, and Duncan Snidal served as the board of advisers for the project. Their insights were invaluable. Franklin I. Gamwell, dean of the Divinity School at the University of Chicago, was supportive throughout. William George was generous with his time in helping with the preparations for each session. Bill's knowledge of international relations and Christian ethics also enhanced the seminar discussions themselves. Robin Lovin's experience in directing similar seminars, and his selfless sharing of his time and insight, saved me from many mistakes. Our conversations on both the substance and form of the seminar were many. Eric Crump helped in editing the article by Trutz Rendtorff.

The Divinity School, the Committee on Public Policy Studies, and the Divinity Students Association, all of the University of Chicago, provided the funding which made the Colloquium possible.

Suzanne Comer, senior editor at Southern Methodist University Press, expressed confidence in the project from its early stages. Because of her blend of professional enthusiasm and efficiency, the results of the Colloquium can be of access to a readership beyond that of the seminar participants. Her efforts have helped to broaden the discussion.

The Colloquium, its participants, and the readers of this volume owe a collective debt to the person who has done most to enliven and deepen the moral-strategic debate from a religious perspective: Paul Ramsey. On February 28, 1988, Mr. Ramsey passed away. He leaves with us a tradition of rigor, intensity, and hope. This collection of essays is dedicated to his memory.

Ethics in the Nuclear Age

Introduction

Two factors have renewed the prospects for ecclesial institutions and scholars in religious studies to participate in the public debate on the possession and use of nuclear weaponry. The first is the impact of the U.S. Catholic bishops' pastoral letter on war and peace, *The Challenge of Peace: God's Promise and Our Response*.[1] Since the writing of this letter, many other denominations have issued their own documents.[2] The second factor is an explicit turn in the discussion among certain strategists and political analysts toward ethical concerns. This is most clearly evidenced by Joseph Nye's book, *Nuclear Ethics*.[3] The developing meeting ground between strategic thought and reflection grounded in religious traditions, then, is ethics. The purpose of this collection of essays is to broaden the range of discussion by drawing together the most recent thought on nuclear ethics by persons trained in religious studies. In doing so, we especially aim to provide a resource both for those who speak for and participate in the church and for strategists who seek to make the moral dimension of the nuclear issue an integral part of their thought.

It is, of course, not new that those in theological ethics or religious studies, both Catholic and Protestant, have turned their attention to the morality of nuclear warfare. John C. Ford's now classic article on obliteration bombing, written just before the nuclear age, set the traditional criteria of proportionality and, especially, noncombatant immunity at the center of just-war thought, where they could be readily retrieved after Hiroshima.[4] John Courtney Murray, Reinhold Niebuhr, and John Bennett all addressed the issue, whether from within or without the just-war tradition.[5] Paul Ramsey sustained the discussion throughout the 1960s with noncombatant immunity as his cornerstone.[6] Ralph Potter and James Childress then each recast and synthesized the criteria, while James T. Johnson contributed historical depth.[7]

It is also the case that religious officials and institutions have issued statements concerning the use and possession of nuclear weapons. The many documents emerging from Protestant denominations and councils are too diverse to summarize here.[8] There are lines of continuity in the Roman Catholic tradition, however, which indicate that the publication of *The Challenge of Peace* is far from being an utter novelty.[9] The Christmas messages of Pius XII, the first pope of the nuclear age, set the critique of nuclear weaponry firmly within the just-war tradition. John XXIII's *Pacem in Terris* of 1963 retains the just-war framework but dramatically shifts the assessment of nuclear weapons: they are now considered to be qualitatively rather than merely quantitatively distinct from conventional arms. *The Pastoral Constitution on the Church in the Modern World (Gaudium et Spes)* of the Second Vatican Council continues this development in thought while granting a wider range to the exercise of personal conscience. *The Challenge of Peace* explicitly identifies *Gaudium et Spes* as its foundational document.[10]

What then accounts for the impact of the bishops' letter? The reasons are several. Certainly timing plays a role. The bishops themselves begin by quoting the Second Vatican Council's statement, "The whole human race faces a moment of supreme crisis in its advance toward maturity." This crisis includes a "new moment" in the public's "awareness of the danger of the nuclear arms race." But public awareness ebbs and flows. Indeed, one task of the church is to work to sustain public attention on crucial issues. A second element in the bishops' success is the sheer force of the fact that they are the institutional representatives of over fifty million Catholic Americans. This gives them reasonable confidence—a sociologically based confidence in addition to that grounded philosophically in natural law—that in speaking to the faithful, they can also address all other U.S. citizens.[11] Still, simple demographic weight, regardless of its theoretical support, grants only an initial hearing.

Perduring engagement in discourse between religionists and strategists depends upon the former doing what the bishops do well: to present an argument around a core set of values that is persuasive from a strategic point of view. It is for this reason that political analysts from Bundy to Wohlstetter feel themselves obliged to respond to the bishops.[12] Timing and the fact that the bishops institutionally represent the moral dimension of the nuclear debate are indeed crucial—these keys, especially the latter, are what individual ethicists often lack. But the success of the bishops is due to their prudential use of these factors to bring public attention to a moral-strategic argument. Lasting influence on public discussion of the issue on the part of the bishops rests on how well they make their case. Previous ecclesiastical documents tend to either refrain from the particulars of policy, in the case of Catholicism, and thus not make a *full* argument, or else simply present a list of policy resolutions, in the case of Protestantism, with perhaps a theological "preface" tacked on.[13]

In the midseventies, this begins to change with the statements of the U.S. Catholic hierarchy, culminating in the 1983 pastoral letter. *The Challenge of Peace* combines an extended interpretation of the Christian moral tradition with a reading of the critical features of contemporary political society and technology—the "signs of the times"—to forge a cogent argument. One part of the overall aim of the present collection of articles is to aid in the maintenance of this high level of reflection as a resource for further ecclesiastical deliberation, especially given the fact that the rapid pace of new technological developments requires ongoing attentiveness to the nuclear issue.[14] Most of the contributors have been official witnesses or consultants in the writing process of church documents.

Given the impact of the pastoral letter and the subsequent response by strategists, it is tempting to assume that the initiative rests solely with the bishops. But there are signs to the contrary. With the important exception of the literature coming out of the Carnegie Council on Ethics and International Affairs (formerly the Council on Religion and International Affairs), the ethical content of various strategic alternatives set forth prior to 1980 is primarily implicit, making inferential analysis necessary to render it explicit.[15] This begins to change, however, as exemplified in writings issuing from some of the faculty at Harvard University. In 1981, Stanley Hoffmann published *Duties beyond Borders: On the Limits and Possibilities of Ethical International Politics,* where he poses two questions: Can moral considerations constitute an integral dimension in the choices of statecraft? If so, how? He holds for the affirmative on the first question. On the second, he rejects both purely deontological and utilitarian options in arguing that the ethics of the political decision maker ought to be one which blends attention to proper ends, means, and principles with a sober reading of the realities of international conflict. Hoffmann then addresses, in turn, the specific issues of the use of force, human rights, distributive justice, and world order. In the first of these, he rejects just-war thought as being dated and inapplicable, but then virtually reconstructs it, adding the category of *jus ante et contra bellum* to the traditional *jus in bello* and *jus ad bellum* with regard to nuclear weapons.[16]

In 1983, Hoffmann joined with several of his colleagues, including Nye, to form the "Harvard Nuclear Study Group," and he wrote *Living with Nuclear Weapons.* In the main, the book attempts to present a straightforward account of the current political and technological state of affairs and of the available alternatives. So Harvard president Derek Bok wrote in the foreword, "We all need to ask and to understand the following important questions: First, what is the nature of our nuclear predicament? Second, what nuclear weaponry exists and why? Third, what can be done?" But in an important, if short, section, they argue for moral restraints on strategy in raising a fourth question: "What Should Be Done?"[17] Here, they use the early drafts of the bishops' letter as a framework for their own reply, but it is clearly not a reply *to* the bishops. The impetus for the section comes from their own reasoning, which places obligations on the state to protect both national sovereignty and the lives of innocent people. National security, which at the present time involves the possession of nuclear weapons, is itself a desirable but limited moral goal, circumscribed by the risks such possession and potential use bring to human life.

Three years later, Joseph Nye, professor of government and former deputy to the undersecretary of state for security assistance under President Carter, published *Nuclear Ethics.* Like Hoffmann, he rejects both Bentham's utilitarian calculus and Kant's categorical imperative as exclusive guides to the moral behavior of representatives of the state in foreign affairs.[18] Instead, he offers a "three-dimensional ethics" which combines considerations—similar to Hoffmann's mix of principles, means, and ends—of motives, means, and consequences. Nye then brings these moral criteria to bear on contemporary political and technological circumstances to construct a nuclear ethics. Bryan Hehir details Nye's position in the first chapter of the present volume.

The publication of *The Challenge of Peace* brought these and other political analysts into fuller discussion with ethical reflection grounded in religious tradition. The present collection of essays seeks to sustain and advance this nascent dialogue.

Although the authors of the articles in this volume are far from full agreement on the moral status of the possession and potential use of nuclear weapons, certain critical perceptions of the issue appear and reappear, with varying emphasis, as leitmotifs throughout the collection.

The first and most dominant is that the particular problematic of deterrence is not simply a quandary which will readily resolve itself if persons use the "correct" mode of moral reasoning, set of principles, and assessment of the facts. The present situation of deterrence produces deeper tensions—if not outright antinomies—in moral theory, political philosophy, and ecclesiology. Stresses in moral reasoning arise due to the divergence in deterrence between intention (to avoid nuclear war) and action (the development and deployment of nuclear missiles), and the resultant inability for either utilitarian calculus or deductive entailment to provide a satisfactory response (Hollenbach, Miller, Yoder, Johnson, Langan, and Whitmore). This has led some thinkers, Michael Walzer the most prominent among them, to argue for "supreme emergency," a situation where considerations of the necessity to preserve one's own civilization override the moral rules of war. The mutual possession and the threat to use nuclear weapons is, for Walzer, a state of permanent supreme emergency.[19] Deterrence strains democratic political theory because once one argues, as the bishops do, that there is virtually no acceptable *use* of the weapons, then the vast majority of the populace must remain ignorant of this "bluff" policy in order for it to remain convincing, thus undermining the idea of an open society (Yoder and Miller). Tensions form in ecclesiology when church officials speak to policy particulars on an issue where, due to the problems with moral reasoning and the diversity of opinion, the possibility of a definitive response is nil. They risk adding to whatever confusion may already exist in the public discussion. The general consensus of the authors is that the bishops earn their way into the debate because they argue well and do not try to overextend their *ecclesiastical* authority. Their *public* authority rests on the quality of their argument (Hollenbach, Yoder, and Whitmore).[20]

The second major theme develops when the perplexities of the problem of deterrence turn critical attention toward the new technologies as possible moral and strategic alternatives to current policy options (Johnson). This shift mirrors the movement of the broader public debate with regard to the moral status of SDI and the relatively small (fractional megatonnage) and accurate (low-CEP) nuclear weaponry.

The structure of the present book builds around the twin issues of deterrence and the possible alternatives as reflecting the state of the moral-strategic debate in religious studies. These are framed within our concern to further the dialogue between the strategists and the churches. Bryan Hehir initiates the collection with an overview of the ethical reasoning of selected strategists. Richard B. Miller, David Hollenbach, and John Howard Yoder then address the problematic of deterrence. James T. Johnson assesses the new technologies. John Langan and Trutz Rendtorff contribute important critiques of the issues in West Germany as counterpoints to the U.S. discussion. Finally, Duane K. Friesen and Todd Whitmore each raise the question of how religious institutions will have to understand and reformulate the inherited tradition in order to adequately address the problem of the possibility of nuclear warfare.

Resting behind the entire project is the conviction that in a pluralistically constituted political society, the more institutionally represented and well-articulated perspectives that are involved in something approximating genuine dialogue, the more tempered public action is likely to be.[21] It is contended in some quarters that this is generally true with the exception of religiously grounded reasoning, which tends to lead to extreme action because the motivating principles are nonnegotiable. This book is an argument to the contrary. A particular case in point is that of "supreme emergency." Despite other disagreements in ethics and policy, none of the authors adopt Walzer's transmoral assent to deterrence. Any acceptance of deterrence must be *through* moral approval and therefore conditioned by the constraints of proportionality and discrimination. The articles by Friesen, Hollenbach, Miller, and Rendtorff suggest why this is more than incidental. To suspend all rules of war under the claim of the necessary survival of one's own civilization is, according to deep and perduring strains of the Christian religious and moral tradition, to idolatrously equate that civilization with the kingdom of God. No *human* threat is ever ultimate, and therefore neither should be any human response. We would argue that the distinction between the city of God and the city of humankind—articulated in the bishops' letter as the "already but not yet" status of God's kingdom in history—brings elements of both restraint and possibility to the moral-strategic debate. It is our hope that our writings reflect both of these aspects of the tradition.

Notes

1. National Conference of Catholic Bishops, *The Challenge of Peace: God's Promise and Our Response* (Washington, D.C.: United States Catholic Conference, 1983).
2. See, for instance, United Church of Christ, General Synod 15, *Social Policy Actions,* "Pronouncement Affirming the United Church of Christ as a Just Peace Church" (New

York: UCC Office for Church in Society, 1985); David Wilbanks and Ronald H. Stone, *Presbyterians and Peacemaking: Are We Called to Resistance?* (New York: Advisory Council on Church and Society of the Presbyterian Church [U.S.A.], 1985); United Methodist Council of Bishops, *In Defense of Creation: The Nuclear Crisis and a Just Peace, Foundation Document* (Nashville, Tenn.: Graded Press, 1986); National Association of Evangelicals, *Guidelines: Peace, Freedom and Security Studies* (Wheaton, Ill.: National Association of Evangelicals, 1986); and Committee of Inquiry on the Nuclear Issue, Commission on Peace, Episcopal Diocese of Washington, *The Nuclear Dilemma: A Christian Search for Understanding* (Cincinnati, Ohio: Forward Movement Publications, 1987).

3. Joseph S. Nye, Jr., *Nuclear Ethics* (New York: Free Press, 1986).

4. John C. Ford, "The Morality of Obliteration Bombing," *Theological Studies* 5 (September 1944): 261–309. Ford continued his analysis of warfare in the nuclear era. See "The Hydrogen Bombing of Cities," in William J. Nagle, ed., *Morality and Modern Warfare* (Baltimore, Md.: Helicon Press, 1960), 98–103.

5. John Courtney Murray, "Remarks on the Moral Problem of War," *Theological Studies* 20 (March 1959): 40–61; and *Morality and Modern War* (New York: Council on Religion and International Affairs, 1959). Reinhold Niebuhr, "The Atomic Bomb" and "The Hydrogen Bomb," in D. B. Robertson, ed., *Love and Justice: Selections from the Shorter Writings of Reinhold Niebuhr* (Philadelphia: Westminster Press, 1957), 232–37. John C. Bennett, "Moral Urgencies in the Nuclear Context," in John C. Bennett, ed., *Nuclear Weapons and the Conflict of Conscience* (New York: Charles Scribner's Sons, 1962), 93–121.

6. Paul Ramsey, *War and the Christian Conscience: How Shall Modern War Be Conducted Justly?* (Durham, N.C.: Duke University Press, 1961); *The Limits of Nuclear War: Thinking about the Do-Able and the Un-Doable* (New York: Council on Religion and International Affairs, 1963); *Again the Justice of Deterrence* (New York: Council on Religion and International Affairs, 1965); and *The Just War: Force and Political Responsibility* (New York: Charles Scribner's Sons, 1968). For commentary on Ramsey's work, see James T. Johnson and David H. Smith, eds., *Love and Society: Essays in the Ethics of Paul Ramsey* (Missoula, Mont.: American Academy of Religion and Scholars Press, 1974).

7. Ralph Potter, *War and Moral Discourse* (Richmond, Va.: John Knox Press, 1969); and "The Moral Logic of War," *McCormick Quarterly* 23 (May 1970): 203–33. James F. Childress, "Just War Criteria," in Thomas A. Shannon, ed., *War or Peace? The Search for New Answers* (Maryknoll, N.Y.: Orbis Books, 1980), 40–58. James T. Johnson, *Ideology, Reason, and the Limitation of War* (Princeton: Princeton University Press, 1975); *Just War Tradition and the Restraint of War: A Moral and Historical Inquiry* (Princeton: Princeton University Press, 1981); and *The Quest for Peace: Three Moral Traditions in Western Cultural History* (Princeton: Princeton University Press, 1987).

8. For a good overview of the documents issued by U.S. churches, see Donald L. Davidson, *Nuclear Weapons and the American Churches: Ethical Positions on Modern Warfare* (Boulder, Colo.: Westview Press, 1983). For excerpts of both Roman Catholic and Protestant documents dating back to 1976, see Robert Heyer, ed., *Nuclear Disarmament: Key Statements of Popes, Bishops, Councils and Churches* (New York: Paulist Press, 1982). Perhaps the best written of the Protestant documents from the perspective of theological attentiveness and sophistication is "The Relation of the Church to the War in Light of the Christian Faith," commissioned by the Federal Council of Churches of Christ in America and chaired by Robert Lowry Calhoun in 1943. The "Calhoun commission," as it is more commonly called, included John Bennett, Roland Bainton, and both H. Richard and Reinhold Niebuhr among its members. James Gustafson discusses the similarities between

this document and *The Challenge of Peace* in "The Bishops' Pastoral Letter: A Theological Ethical Analysis," *Criterion* 23 (Spring 1984): 5–10. The doctrinal section of the commission report is reprinted in John H. Leith, *Creeds of the Churches* (Atlanta, Ga.: John Knox Press, 1982), 522–54.

9. William Au develops in detail the antecedents to the bishops' letter in *The Cross, the Flag, and the Bomb: American Catholics Debate War and Peace, 1960–1983* (Westport, Conn.: Greenwood Press, 1985). For collections of the documents, see Joseph Gremillion, ed., *The Gospel of Peace and Justice: Catholic Social Teaching since Pope John* (Maryknoll, N.Y.: Orbis Books, 1976); Heyer, *Nuclear Disarmament;* David J. O'Brien and Thomas A. Shannon, eds., *Renewing the Earth: Catholic Documents on Peace, Justice and Liberation* (Garden City, N.Y.: Image Books, 1977); and J. Brian Benestead and Francis J. Butler, eds., *Quest for Justice: A Compendium of Statements of the United States Catholic Bishops on the Political and Social Order 1966–1980* (Washington, D.C.: United States Catholic Conference, 1981).

10. See V. Yzermans, ed., *Major Addresses of Pius XII,* vol. 2 (St. Paul, Minn.: North Central Publishing Co., 1961); *Pacem in Terris,* pars. 109–19, 126–29; *The Pastoral Constitution on the Church in the Modern World (Gaudium et Spes),* pars. 77–82; and *The Challenge of Peace,* par. 7.

11. *The Challenge of Peace,* par. 1, from *Gaudium et Spes,* par. 77; *Gaudium et Spes,* pars. 125–38, 4, and 16–19.

12. McGeorge Bundy, "The Bishops and the Bomb," *New York Review of Books* (June 16, 1983), 1–6. Albert Wohlstetter, "Bishops, Statesmen and Other Strategists on the Bombing of Innocents," *Commentary* (June 1983), 15–35; and "Morality and Deterrence: Wohlstetter and Critics," *Commentary* (December 1983), 13–22. For a thorough commentary on the bishops' letter carried out by a political analyst, see James E. Dougherty, *The Bishops and Nuclear Weapons: The Catholic Pastoral Letter on War and Peace* (Hamden, Conn.: Archon Books, 1984).

13. For a critique of the Protestant tendency, see Paul Ramsey, *Who Speaks for the Church?* (Nashville: Abingdon Press, 1967).

14. For analyses of the new technologies, see James E. Dougherty, "Technological Developments and the Evaluation of War," in William V. O'Brien and John Langan, S.J., *The Nuclear Dilemma and the Just War Tradition* (Lexington, Mass.: Lexington Books, 1986), 81–128; and Peter deLeon, *The Altered Strategic Environment: Toward the Year 2000* (Lexington, Mass.: Lexington Books, 1987).

15. See J. Bryan Hehir's "Ethics and Strategy: The Views of Selected Strategists" in this volume. Hehir notes the exceptions of Nitze and Brennan as strategists who on occasion did do ethical analysis.

16. Stanley Hoffmann, *Duties beyond Borders: On the Limits and Possibilities of Ethical International Politics* (Syracuse, N.Y.: Syracuse University Press, 1981), 1, 10, 30, 45–93.

17. Albert Carnsdale, Paul Doty, Stanley Hoffmann, Samuel P. Huntington, Joseph S. Nye, Jr., and Scott D. Sagan, *Living with Nuclear Weapons* (New York: Bantam Books, 1983), ix, 243–49.

18. Nye, *Nuclear Ethics,* 16–20.

19. Michael Walzer, *Just and Unjust Wars: A Moral Argument with Historical Illustrations* (New York: Basic Books, 1977), 251–83.

20. J. Bryan Hehir also holds that the bishops earn their way into the public debate through the quality of their argument. See "Moral Aspects of the Nuclear Arms Debate: The Contribution of the U.S. Catholic Bishops," in Robert C. Johansen, ed., *The Nuclear*

Arms Debate: Ethical and Political Implications (Princeton: Center of International Studies, 1983), 34–36.

21. Both Hehir and Langan in other contexts have argued that the bishops' letter brought the moral dimension to the strategic-military debate. Ibid., 22–24; John Langan, S.J., in the introduction to O'Brien and Langan, *Nuclear Dilemma,* 7–9.

I · STRATEGY

1 • Ethics and Strategy: The Views of Selected Strategists

J. BRYAN HEHIR

The purpose of this paper is to examine the ethical arguments of selected nuclear strategists. The topic itself is a product of the changing state of the nuclear debate in the 1980s. While a substantial corpus of moral argument on nuclear policy had been developed by philosophers and theologians from the early 1960s through the early 1980s, these materials did not play a significant role in the writings of political analysts or strategic thinkers.

The 1980s have produced several changes in the intellectual and political shape of the nuclear policy debate. A quite visible change has been the democratization of policy discussion well beyond the standard participants of those in the government, in think tanks, and at a few major universities. A less publicly recognized change has been the fissures created in the policy community about the direction nuclear strategy should take. From proposals for "no first use" of nuclear weapons, to proposals for resurrecting "defensive systems," to vigorous dissent—within the policy community—on the Reagan administration's negotiating positions at the Reykjavik summit and the Intermediate Nuclear Forces (INF) negotiations in Geneva, there has been a shattering of the policy consensus that previously undergirded debate on specific tactics in the elite policy community. Finally, the 1980s have brought the significance of moral concerns about nuclear policy to a central place in both the popular debate about nuclear weapons and in the policy community.[1]

It is this change in the place of ethical argument in the policy debate which has moved political and strategic commentators to address ethical issues in their own writings. In response to this development, this paper will have three objectives: (1) to sketch the framework of ethical argument which has developed in the last twenty-five years; (2) to examine the writings of selected strategists in light of that framework; and (3) to comment on the present state and future direction of the ethics and strategy debate.

Ethics and Strategy: The Basic Positions

In the last twenty-five years three basic positions on the ethics of nuclear strategy were set forth. In addition to these three, the pastoral letter of the Catholic bishops, *The Challenge of Peace,* argued a position which reflected earlier views but could not be totally identified with any one of them. I will sketch the logic and conclusions of these four positions.

All of the positions examined here are rooted in a just-war (or just-defense) ethic.[2] They all accept the moral legitimacy of some use of force in international affairs, but they all assert that any morally legitimate use of force must be a limited use. The principles of limitation (presuming a just cause) are discrimination (or noncombatant immunity) and proportionality. The fundamental question the traditional just-war ethic has to address is whether nuclear weapons and nuclear strategy are inherently and irretrievably in conflict with the classical principles of limitation on the use of force. In addressing this basic question, the ethical arguments surveyed here have focused on two issues: whether nuclear weapons could be used in a morally justifiable way and whether the strategic preparations for use and the threat/intention to use nuclear forces in a strategy of deterrence could be justified.

Justifying Deterrence: Paul Ramsey and William O'Brien

The first position argues that classical just-war categories can be used to set moral limits on the use of nuclear weapons and to shape deterrence posture in a morally justifiable fashion. This position has been developed by Paul Ramsey in the 1960s and William O'Brien in the 1970s.[3]

The foundation of the moral argument is the conviction of continuity in the moral problem of war in the pre- and post-nuclear ages. While acknowledging empirical difference between nuclear weapons and other forms of force, these authors do not admit a qualitative difference in the nuclear question. The question today, as in the past, is how to set moral limits to the forces available to statespersons.

With this traditional definition of the moral task, they seek to shape force structure and targeting doctrine in ways that meet standards of noncombatant immunity and proportionality. Ramsey, for example, developed detailed arguments in the 1960s about the moral possibilities of limited nuclear war, setting forth the conditions of both just cause and permissible means which could be used in the European theatre. At the strategic level Ramsey found Robert McNamara's "No Cities" speech at Ann Arbor in 1962 to be the kind of initiative moralists should support. William O'Brien in both the 1970s and 1980s follows the general direction of Ramsey's argument, although he is both more cautious about prospects for keeping nuclear use limited and more willing to treat noncombatant immunity as a rule of thumb rather than a nonnegotiable moral principle.

This position first establishes the limits of the morally permissible in terms of nuclear weapons use, then argues for a deterrent that threatens only morally acceptable strikes. In military terms this is a strictly defined counterforce position at both the theatre and strategic policy levels.

In support of this counterforce use policy, Ramsey proposed a deterrence posture based on three morally acceptable threats: (1) deterrence based on disproportionate combatant damage; (2) deterrence based on disproportionate collateral damage; and (3) deterrence based on the inherently ambiguous operational capabilities of nuclear weapons.

The position of justifying deterrence faces two sets of problems. First, from the strategist's perspective it must confront all the standard criticisms made of the counterforce position. The objections include the danger (in spite of good moral intentions) of conveying a first-strike intent to one's adversary; of increasing the incentive to preempt in crisis situations; and of opening an endless spiral of ever larger defense budgets in pursuit of a credible counterforce posture. Second, from the moralist's perspective the Ramsey-O'Brien position must answer two sets of questions. On the one hand, the risk of escalation beyond carefully tailored limited use leads many to question whether the risk is proportionate. On the other, the problem of colocation of military targets leads many (strategists and ethicists) to see the counterforce targeting of these installations as a distinction with little moral difference from direct attacks on civilians. (There is some difference in terms of moral theory, but it may not render the attacks morally permissible.)

It is precisely these kinds of objections to the Ramsey-O'Brien position that have led other moralists to reject deterrence.

Rejecting Deterrence: Walter Stein and Anthony Kenny

Stein and Kenny are convinced that the only permissible moral position is the rejection of deterrence. This position of "nuclear pacifism" found initial expression in Stein's anthology, *Nuclear Weapons and the Christian Conscience* (1961), a position recently reaffirmed by Kenny in

The Logic of Deterrence (1985).[4] These two versions differ both in moral argument and in their empirical assessment of the nuclear reality, but they arrive at the same conclusion on deterrence.

The Stein volume, an anthology of Catholic philosophers, essentially argued that any use of nuclear weapons would certainly violate the principle of proportionality and probably violate noncombatant immunity. From this judgment the several authors moved to an evaluation of deterrence in a line of argument which was as stark in its conclusion as it was simple in its logic. Since nuclear weapons are inherently disproportionate, it is wrong to use them; since it is wrong to use them, it is wrong to intend to use them. Since nuclear deterrence requires the intention to do what one threatens, the strategy is immoral.

Embedded in this argument is a moral theory of intentionality which would take an essay to describe and defend. Although not exclusively Catholic in content, it has been used especially in a range of Catholic arguments. The theory declares that to intend to do evil is to be morally implicated in the evil even if the intention is never implemented. There is, of course, a difference of degree between intending evil and doing evil, but both carry moral significance.

This notion of intentionality is central to Kenny's argument, but his position differs from Stein's in one regard. The authors of the Stein volume, examining nuclear weapons in the early 1960s, could point easily to the indiscriminate character of the nuclear arsenal. Kenny is aware of those technological changes which made nuclear weapons less "dirty" and indiscriminate. Hence, Kenny acknowledges that some use of nuclear weapons might meet just-war criteria. But he argues that the risk of escalation is too high to justify discrete instances of use. Regarding deterrence, it is again the risk of escalation which is decisive; the superpower arsenals in aggregate terms clearly go beyond what could be legitimately used, and Kenny is of the opinion that a Soviet response to even a limited use of nuclear weapons would push both superpowers up the escalation ladder to unjustifiable warfare.

For Stein of the 1960s and Kenny of the 1980s, therefore, nuclear weapons move beyond the legitimate use of force. Both authors can only advise dissent from deterrence as a policy position and as a personal choice. Such a position faces both political and ethical objections. Politically, the position is described as at best purist, at worst irrelevant. Such a charge may miss the political weight which large-scale conscientious objection might have, but the charge does point to the way in which the Stein-Kenny argument can be respected within the policy debate, but not utilized in that context. Ethically, the critique of the Stein-Kenny position is that it isolates the theme of intention and gives it too much moral weight. In Joseph Nye's words the stress on intentionality "is too simple an approach to strategic action to be able to capture the situation of deterrence."[5]

Tolerating Deterrence: Michael Walzer

In the 1960s one could choose between Stein and Ramsey; in the 1970s Michael Walzer developed a distinct position in *Just and Unjust Wars*. Walzer is fully cognizant of the moral problems associated with deterrence: "Anyone committed to the distinction between combatants and noncombatants is bound to be appalled by the spectre of destruction evoked, and purposely evoked in deterrence theory."[6]

Indeed Walzer's judgment on the use of nuclear weapons is as absolute as that of Stein and his colleagues in the 1960s. In spite of changes in accuracy and yield, Walzer finds nuclear weapons unusable: "They are the first of mankind's technological innovations that are simply not encompassable within the familiar moral world."[7]

But the *threat* to use such weapons, even against civilians, is a different moral issue for Walzer. Following a moral argument used to justify British bombing policy in 1940–42, he describes the nuclear deterrence relationship as a situation of "supreme emergency." The phrase refers to a condition where a mortal threat is lodged against a community and the danger is imminent. When both characteristics are present, the political community and its leaders are brought "under the rule of necessity (and necessity knows no rules)."[8] In the nuclear age,

> supreme emergency has become a permanent condition. Deterrence
> is a way of coping with that condition, and though it is a bad way,
> there may well be no other that is practical in a world of sovereign
> and suspicious states. We threaten evil in order not to do it, and
> the doing of it would be so terrible that the threat seems in compari-
> son to be morally defensible.[9]

In this argument Walzer stretches both empirical and ethical principles to the breaking point. Having acknowledged that intentionality is a central part of the ethical problem of deterrence, he overrides its claims by justifying deterrence threats which (he argues) violate the principle of noncombatant immunity. In the empirical order, Walzer so divides use doctrine and deterrence doctrine that the credibility of deterrence is endangered. At the same time it should be acknowledged that some versions of strategic theory suffer the same tension.

These three "types" of the ethics of deterrence remain today as the framework for assessing strategic policy. Variations exist but they do not appear as logically distinct positions. One variation which has particularly attracted the attention of strategists is the pastoral letter of the Catholic bishops.

Conditional Acceptance of Deterrence: The Challenge of Peace

The pastoral letter was, like the other positions examined in this paper, a classical just-war assessment of the nuclear age. In contrast to Ramsey's position, the bishops stressed the qualitative difference of the pre- and post-nuclear ages. In contrast to Stein's position, they did not condemn deterrence or counsel simply an ethic of resistance to nuclear strategy. At first glance the position of the pastoral letter has some affinity with Walzer, but differences in conclusions and in styles of reasoning are evident.

On the question of the use of nuclear weapons, the bishops distinguish three cases of possible use.[10] The moral argument runs from an absolute prohibition to a carefully circumscribed possibility of use. The pastoral letter rules out absolutely directly intended attacks on civilian centers. The U.S. letter follows the Second Vatican Council in condemning such strikes and it adds a specific note by ruling them out even if U.S. cities are hit first.

The U.S. letter took a position in favor of a "no first use" pledge by NATO. The rationale supporting the position involved two dimensions. On one hand, the bishops argued that a special moral responsibility is involved in taking the world into nuclear war; the burden of proof to justify such a step falls on the initiator, and the pastoral letter gave no support to a first-use policy. On the other hand, the bishops were aware that this proscription cuts right across existing NATO policy. But the thrust of the pastoral letter is to build a barrier against early, easy, or preemptive use of nuclear weapons. The "no first use" prohibition is part of that overall design, as was their stated willingness to support some increased spending on conventional forces.

The pastoral letter moved from first use to a third case "limited nuclear war." Here the letter took a less absolute position than it did on countercivilian strikes and a less definite position than it took on first use. The argument on second-strike limited use involved raising a series of questions about the possibilities of limiting such an exchange, and then clearly placing the burden of proof again on those who would justify such strikes because they could be limited. The bishops are radically skeptical of the empirical claim, but they do not move to a moral prohibition of all use of nuclear weapons (as Stein does) because of their empirical skepticism.

In light of these three cases of use the pastoral letter considered the strategy of deterrence. The judgment on deterrence is what the bishops call "strictly conditioned moral acceptance." The phrase places two kinds of restraint on the strategy of deterrence. The first is "temporal" in nature; it ties the justification for deterrence to an understanding that it be used as a framework for moving to a different basis of security among nations. This temporal assessment means that the "direction" of deterrence policy has moral significance—are steps being taken to move away from this fragile, paradoxical basis for interstate relations or is the direction of policy simply reinforcing the present state of affairs?

The second restraint concerns the "character" of the deterrent. The strictly conditioned justification of the deterrent rests upon its role of "preventing the use of nuclear weapons or other actions which could lead directly to a nuclear exchange."[11] The point here is to limit the role of nuclear deterrence to a very specific function in world affairs; the posture of deterrence is not to be used to pursue goals other than preventing nuclear war. To give specific content to this limited concept of deterrence the bishops make a series of concrete proposals:

The bishops oppose: (1) extending deterrence to a variety of war-fighting strategies; (2) a quest for strategic superiority; (3) any blurring of the distinction between nuclear and conventional weapons; and (4) the deployment of weapons with "hard-target-kill" capability.

The bishops support: (1) immediate, bilateral, verifiable agreements to halt the testing, production, and deployment of new nuclear systems; (2) negotiating strategies aimed at deep cuts in superpower arsenals; (3) conclusion of a comprehensive test ban treaty; and (4) strengthening of command and control systems for nuclear weapons.[12]

The pastoral letter generated an enormous amount of commentary while it was being written and after its publication. It has encountered two kinds of criticisms. From the perspective of ethical analysis two different types of arguments are made against the pastoral letter. One is that the letter's failure to rule out all use of nuclear weapons is not supported by convincing evidence that limited use is possible. A second critique argues that the letter's logic clearly should have led the bishops to a position of nuclear pacifism. The conclusion of these two positions is the same, but the first criticizes the bishops' use of empirical data, the second their failure to abide by the moral logic of their arguments.

From the strategists' perspective two different criticisms are made. One is that by stressing the limits to be placed on nuclear weapons the bishops have stripped deterrence of a credible threat. The other is that the bishops' endorsement of specific policy proposals does not constitute an internally coherent policy.

The range of commentators on the pastoral letter extended beyond the community of those who had previously written on the ethics of strategy. All of the strategists examined in the next section addressed the pastoral letter explicitly, and implicitly they were drawn into the wider debate sketched above.

Selected Strategists: A Spectrum of Views

In assessing the views of strategists a different approach is needed. These authors are often less explicit in using ethical categories and moral principles, even when their purpose is to address the ethics of strategy. To evaluate these authors usually requires a process of rendering explicit a mode of moral reasoning often embedded in a political-strategic argument. In this section I will use three questions to probe the ethics of the strategists: (1) What are their ethical concerns? (2) How do they relate ethics to political-strategic analysis? (3) What policy prescriptions do they advance?

Albert Wohlstetter: Usable Nuclear Weapons

In any history of nuclear strategy Albert Wohlstetter's article "The Delicate Balance of Terror," published in *Foreign Affairs* in 1959, is always cited as a canonical text. By illustrating the vulnerability of the U.S. retaliatory force and by stressing the fragility of the nuclear balance, Wohlstetter catalyzed the effort that led to the dispersal of nuclear forces, the development of silo-based missiles, and the deployment of U.S. nuclear striking forces in a "triad" of land-based and sea-based missiles along with bombers. Wohlstetter, a prolific author and veteran consultant to U.S. administrations on nuclear matters, chose the occasion of the pastoral letter to reenter the nuclear debate, this time focusing on the intersection of ethics and strategic doctrine. In an extended essay, "Bishops, Statesmen and Other Strategists on the Bombing of Innocents,"[13] Wohlstetter manifests a central concern of his effort. It is to do well what, in his view, the Catholic bishops did poorly: to evaluate and redirect Western nuclear strategy in light of the principle of discrimination. While Wohlstetter's article has none of the philosophical-theological underpinning of the noncombatant immunity principle found in Paul Ramsey's articles, he stands in the direct lineage of Ramsey's work. His ethical critique of existing strategy and his criticisms of other efforts of moral analysis—including both the bishops and Michael Walzer—are that they give lip service to noncombatant immunity, but either tolerate threats to violate the principle or use the principle to advocate (nuclear) pacifism. Wohlstetter, basing his argument on a standard interpretation of the discrimination principle and an equally traditional extension of it to rule out the threat/intention to strike civilians, will neither justify such threats nor disarm the West.

Neither conclusion is necessary because the imperatives of enlightened strategic planning and traditional moral guidance coincide in the 1980s. What makes this fortuitous convergence possible is technological change.

Today, the combination of increasingly accurate missiles equipped with miniaturized nuclear warheads makes the prospect of discrete, discriminate attacks, even over great distances, a real possibility. Hence, Wohlstetter's critique of the bishops is that they had the right moral principle (discrimination), but they took the wrong technical advice, thereby producing greater confusion in the public debate on nuclear policy:

> Only some widely prevalent but shallow evasions and self-befuddlements, and not any deep moral dilemma or basic paradox, force us to threaten the annihilation of civilians in order to prevent nuclear or conventional war. The bishops are clear about rejecting the actual use of nuclear weapons to kill innocents. About threats to kill innocents, they are much less clear. Their obscurity mirrors an uneasy area of darkness at the core of establishment views.[14]

The darkness in the secular and religious establishments can be dispelled if it is recognized that the technologies of increasing accuracy and smaller warheads, now waiting to be used, present not only a moral breakthrough but also the most credible deterrent threat to the Soviet Union, and it is the Soviet Union that must be deterred.

Wohlstetter finds the ethics and strategy debate beset by two misconceptions which prevent it from recognizing the dual blessing conferred by recent technology. The moralists seem to base their understanding of the indiscriminate destructiveness of nuclear weapons on data more relevant to weapons of the 1950s. Since that time, "the prospects of hitting only what one is aiming at have increased by several orders of magnitude."[15] This dissolves the old dilemma about nuclear use and creates a moral responsibility for the West to develop the more discriminate weapons.

The misconception of the strategists is holding on to the idea that assured destruction of Soviet society is a credible threat to the Soviets, when it is clear that they "value their military power, on the evidence, more than the lives of bystanders."[16]

The consequence of this double mistake is that in the newly revived nuclear debate of the 1980s some of the moralists and some of the strategists reinforce each other's error. The moralists rule out any use of nuclear weapons ("use never") and the strategists hold that "deterrence only" (based on mutual assured destruction) is an adequate strategic posture.

In contrast Wohlstetter urges a thorough recasting of the reigning strategic wisdom, using as his principle of reconstruction a commitment to protection of noncombatants. In policy terms, Wohlstetter advocates using the full range of new technologies to improve the precision of both nuclear weapons and conventional weapons. The effect of this would be to enhance extended deterrence in the European theatre, and to provide a strategic striking force that not only will put at risk Soviet hard targets, but also will provide a morally defensible second-strike posture. Wohlstetter would bolster a more accurate nuclear striking force with expanded conventional forces, and he seems to support defensive systems deployed for purposes of damage limitation.

In brief, he seeks a usable nuclear force, one which can pass the moral tests of discrimination and proportionality, and which a U.S. president would not refrain from using because it would begin a nuclear holocaust.

Wohlstetter's ethical-strategic position opposes both the "use never" of some moralists and the "deterrence only" of some strategists.

McGeorge Bundy: Existential Deterrence

The position McGeorge Bundy espoused in the early 1980s embodies much of what Wohlstetter opposes in the contemporary nuclear discussion. Bundy has combined a distinguished academic career with his experience as national security adviser in the Kennedy and Johnson administrations. Beginning with an article in *Foreign Affairs* in 1969,[17] and continuing through the 1980s, Bundy has developed a conception of the uses and limits of the nuclear arsenal that moves in a very different direction from Wohlstetter. From the 1969 article, which argued that nuclear weapons should do no less than deter, but could not be expected to do more than deter, to his role in the "no first use" article in 1982,[18] to his advocacy of existential deterrence in 1983, Bundy has sought to redefine and redirect U.S. policy on deterrence.

In this process, Bundy has been less explicit than Wohlstetter in his address to the ethics of nuclear strategy. He first engaged the ethical issues in a commentary on *The Challenge of Peace,* using the occasion of the letter to set forth the idea of existential deterrence.

It is clear that Bundy believes the best—perhaps only—way to adhere to the traditional moral principles of warfare in the nuclear age is to prevent nuclear war in any form. Hence, there is no detailed discussion of how to set limits on nuclear use as one finds in Ramsey and Wohlstetter. Bundy is pessimistic about such limits in the nuclear age (although, as we shall see, he does address the topic in his own way). Bundy's pivotal point is to distinguish nuclear strategy and nuclear war from our prenuclear conceptions of strategy and war.

Wohlstetter's overriding moral concern is protecting the principle of discrimination in nuclear planning and execution. Bundy's main moral concern is to drive home the following proposition:

> As long as each side retains survivable strength so that no leader
> can ever suppose that he could "disarm" his opponent completely,
> nuclear war remains an overwhelmingly unattractive proposition
> for both sides. This is the reality from which moralists and po-
> litical analysts must draw the same great conclusion: no to nuclear
> war.[19]

The strategic transposition of this ethical position is the theory of existential deterrence. Bundy begins with the bishops' judgment of "conditional acceptance" of deterrence, adding the gloss that "in our current debates their strict conditions may be more significant than their approval."[20] He then goes on to state the case for existential deterrence:

> The terrible and unavoidable uncertainties in any recourse to nuclear war create what could be called "existential" deterrence, where the function of the adjective is to distinguish this phenomenon from anything based on strategic theories or declared policies or even international commitments. As long as each side has large numbers of thermonuclear weapons that could be used against the opponent, even after the strongest possible preemptive attack, existential deterrence is strong and it rests on uncertainty about what could happen.[21]

Bundy never disparages deterrence; it is indispensable for the foreseeable future. But he has a very specific understanding of its function. By the 1980s Bundy, in addressing the ethical issues more explicitly, made an important qualification of his 1969 position. There he had concluded an analysis of how irrational nuclear war would be with the following statement:

> In the real world of real political leaders—whether here or in the Soviet Union—a decision that would bring even one hydrogen bomb on one city of one's own country would be recognized in advance as a catastrophic blunder; ten bombs on ten cities would be a disaster beyond history; and a hundred bombs on a hundred cities an unthinkable.[22]

In a 1983 address at San Francisco University, Bundy went out of his way to make the following emendation:

> It is now clear that there is every reason for limiting damage to cities in any plan for nuclear retaliation. The minimization of the loss of innocent life is a proper imperative even for capabilities whose main purpose is to deter, not to prevail in war, and I recognize that by offering an illustration based on the loss of cities I may have seemed to contribute to the acceptance of cities as targets which was widespread at the time.[23]

Bundy's position is close to but not identical with the "deterrence only" position Wohlstetter criticized. Bundy's differences with that position show up when he addresses—in more detail than the bishops, but with much less enthusiasm than Wohlstetter and less confidence than Ramsey—the question of second use of nuclear weapons. Bundy's policy prescriptions about nuclear use are grounded in a basic principle: "It must be the object of policy to reduce the number of cases in which we rely on any use of nuclear weapons whatever.[24] In the light of this basic posture Bundy then addresses what to do if deterrence fails.

His policy involves a series of propositions, each designed to move back from the nuclear abyss:

1. *No first use* of nuclear weapons; conventional capabilities should meet a conventional attack.
2. *No second use until* it is clear the West has been attacked by nuclear weapons and the nature of the attack is assessed.
3. Any response to a nuclear attack should be clearly and substantially *smaller* than the initial attack.
4. No "decapitation" strategy for the West, i.e., the objective of Western policy should be to keep the Soviet leadership alive so bargaining can proceed to terminate the nuclear exchange.[25]

These guidelines complement existential deterrence in a policy which is a counterpoint to Wohlstetter's proposals for nuclear strategy. It is difficult to trace Bundy's position to any of the three basic ethical positions. He has developed an analogical position to *The Challenge of Peace*, but there are important differences in the two positions.

Joseph Nye, Jr.: Maxims for Nuclear Strategy

Joseph Nye's book *Nuclear Ethics* is itself a sign of the new stage of the dialogue between ethics and strategy. Nye, a prolific author on political-strategic questions and a former senior official in the Carter administration, has written a careful, informed essay on the moral issues in the nuclear age. Nye develops his argument by reviewing other contributions to the field and then constructing his own position. His position is a revised statement of the just-war ethic, which he usefully renames the just-defense ethic. From his reading in moral philosophy and the just-war tradition, Nye concludes that an adequate policy ethic must test motives, means, and consequences of action.

Nye's basic judgment of deterrence is "conditional acceptance," an evaluation he ties to the U.S. bishops' letter. But Nye's position is not identical with *The Challenge of Peace*. While the ultimate evaluation of deterrence is quite similar, Nye is skeptical of the way the bishops assessed the use of nuclear weapons. The problem both ethicists and strategists face is the "usability dilemma": "Given the existence of some risk of unintended horrible consequences, one should wish to avoid any use of nuclear weapons. But if there is absolutely no possibility of the use of nuclear weapons, or if that is believed to be the case, they will have no deterrent effects."[26] Nye is more willing than the bishops were to specify which use of nuclear weapons would seem to fit the just-defense criteria, and he is much less inclined to support a "no first use" pledge on either ethical or empirical grounds. He divides with Bundy over "no first use," but his conception of what would be justifiable use is closer to Bundy than to Wohlstetter. Nye, therefore, joins some flexibility on use with a narrowly defined conditional assent for deterrence. This framework is then used to provide policy advice in terms of five maxims for the nuclear age.[27]

The maxims are designed to respond to Nye's grid of motives, means, and consequences. Hence, they are

Motives
   1. Self-defense is a just but limited cause.
Means
   2. Never treat nuclear weapons as normal weapons.
   3. Minimize harm to innocent people.
Consequences
   4. Reduce risks to nuclear war in the near term.
   5. Reduce reliance on nuclear weapons over time.

Nye expands his analysis of each maxim, seeking to shape a unified policy. Three points of particular note will situate his position vis-à-vis others analyzed in this paper. Maxim 2 places Nye closer to Bundy than Wohlstetter, closer to the bishops than to Ramsey, but it also must be seen in light of Nye's resolution of the usability paradox. His presumption is to keep the nuclear vs. conventional distinction firm ("never treat"), but he is not prepared to say "never use" or "never use first." The presumption that nuclear weapons are a special case yields to a range of exceptions covering both theatre use of nuclear weapons and selected strategic strikes.

The exceptions to maxim 2 lead to Nye's maxim 3. Nye's formulation is carefully drawn; he wants to respect the principle of discrimination but not be paralyzed by it. His solution, following William O'Brien, is to treat discrimination as a "relative principle."[28] Nye presses the requirements of discrimination quite far; he advocates changes in U.S. targeting doctrine to reduce civilian casualties, and he argues that such changes would be a strategic improvement as well as a moral benefit. But he judges that Ramsey, Wohlstetter, and the Catholic bishops are all too tied to purity on the principle of discrimination, and the result is to drive nuclear strategy in an unproductive search for "clean strikes."

Nye's maxims 4 and 5 reflect the judgment of the pastoral letter that conditional acceptance of deterrence should be joined with movement away from the central role nuclear weapons have played in the superpower relationship and in world politics generally. There can be some tension when one tries to implement both maxim 4 and maxim 5: pursuit of the latter can pose dangers for the former. This is one of the criticisms lodged against President Reagan's SDI program. Analysts worry that this attempt to reduce reliance on nuclear weapons may well raise the risks of an offensive-defensive arms race in the short term.

Zbigniew Brzezinski: The Defensive Option

Zbigniew Brzezinski is aware of the danger cited by critics of the president's proposal, but he finds a hopeful possibility for ethics and for strategy in an offensive-defensive mix. Brzezinski is a veteran contributor to the strategic debate and served as national security adviser in the Carter administration. In a 1986 essay, "The Strategic Implications of Thou Shalt Not Kill,"[29] he addressed the intersection of ethics and strategy. He interprets *The Challenge of Peace* as advocating three criteria for ethical analysis: discrimination, proportionality, and probability of success. Brzezinski then assesses the nuclear relationship of the 1980s in search of a strategic posture which will be militarily credible and ethically acceptable.

Empirically, Brzezinski is impressed by two characteristics of the 1980s. The technological changes of accuracy and miniaturization central to Wohlstetter's position have made nuclear weapons "instruments capable of being employed in a preemptive first strike, designed not so much to destroy the opponent's society as a whole but to eliminate his strategic forces."[30] In addition the Soviets' "massive and ongoing buildup" of their strategic arsenal means they have taken advantage of these technological changes and they could in the future "design an attack that would leave the United States crippled, capable of only a spasmodic, disorganized and strategically aimless response—which would also be attrited by Soviet missile defenses."

Faced with this strategic landscape, Brzezinski evaluates four possible U.S. responses. The general character of his analysis is principally a review of policy options and only obliquely a commentary on the ethics of policy.

He finds reliance on arms control as a principle mode of response in-effective; the president's version of SDI is infeasible in the short to mid term; and a continuing reliance on mutual assured destruction is empirically and ethically objectionable: "Ultimately, the long-run failing of MAD is that it is fundamentally not credible, in addition to raising serious moral questions."[31]

Brzezinski's proposal to meet the criteria of strategic credibility and ethical legitimacy is a combination of "limited strategic defense and limited strategic offense." The proposal signals a new chapter in the ethics and strategy debate, one opened by the president's argument that defensive systems are the answer to the moral dilemma of the nuclear age. Brzezinski is not prepared to advocate the president's moral-strategic policy of the search for perfect defense, but of all the authors surveyed here he takes a defensive option most seriously.

At this point, I can only note the emergence of the defensive proposals as an inevitable part of the ethics and strategy debate. Brzezinski's policy design—which he sets forth and then simply asserts that it meets the bishops' ethical criteria—is only one way the defensive case can be argued. Colin Gray and Keith Payne advocate a plan much closer to the Reagan design for a defense-dominated nuclear age.[32]

Brzezinski wants enough defense to eliminate in Soviet minds the prospect that they could launch a successful first strike on U.S. nuclear forces. He wants enough offensive forces to provide the United States with (1) the capability for a limited (i.e., not disarming) selective first strike on the Soviet Union and (2) a strong second-strike capability. He is careful to stress that both his defensive and offensive forces will be "limited," to put at rest Soviet fears that we seek either an "invulnerable" United States or a disarming first-strike strategy.

Brzezinski's proposal will face both ethical and empirical criticism, because his hopeful vision of an offensive-defensive mix is for others, ethicists and strategists, a nightmare of uncertainty and complexity which many believe will raise the risk of a nuclear mistake in the short term, but will not alleviate the nuclear dilemma in the long run.

Ethics and Strategy: Future Directions

This paper has sketched the same landscape from two perspectives. The first phase of the ethics and strategy debate (1969–80) was dominated by philosophers and theologians. While it is true that some political-strategic analysts and actors such as Donald Brennan[33] and Paul Nitze[34] made contributions to the discussion, they were not known for these writings. The second stage of the debate (the 1980s) has engaged a new range of contributors less versed in technical ethical argument but very interested in grasping the intersection of ethics and strategy. The future discussion of ethics and strategy will draw upon the resources of both stages of the debate which have been traced here. Three arguments which will shape the future will be (1) the place of ethics in strategic analysis; (2) the status of deterrence as a concept and a policy; and (3) the quest to go "beyond deterrence."

The intensified interest in and visibility of ethical analysis in the 1980s brought with it diverse evaluations of the contribution of ethics to the standard strategic analysis. Three positions are visible on this question: ethics as irrelevant; ethics as decisive; and ethics as complementary to strategic discourse.

One perspective is that ethical evaluation is irrelevant, that it adds nothing analytically to our understanding of the strategic choices statespersons face or to the arms control policies which should be pursued. This assessment differs from the "realist" case that war and defense issues are too vital for national security to be subjected to ethical restraints. The critique of "irrelevance" is perfectly willing to have ethics be included in the debate because it is convinced that whatever ethical analysis affirms can be equally well grasped by standard strategic analysis.

The second perspective, ethics as decisive, moves in precisely the opposite direction. It holds that once the "ethically correct" posture is grasped then policy can be set in light of this perspective. This argument for the primacy of ethics as opposed to the irrelevance of ethics can move in different directions. The logic of the Stein-Kenny position is that the identification of an "intention to do evil" embedded in deterrence requires that one withdraw support and/or cooperation from the policy. Wohlstetter displays a similar confidence leading to a contradictory conclusion: discrimination plus technique will dissolve the dilemma of deterrence.

But this focus on an "ethic of means" can be contrasted with a quite different view of the decisiveness of ethics. The second perspective can use an "ethic of ends" to argue that the threat posed by one's adversary (e.g., the threat of communist domination) is so inherently evil that *any* means is a legitimate response to forestall the threat. In both of these examples, one "ethical" insight cuts through the normal complexity of the policy process of balancing a multiplicity of values, objectives, methods, and tactics in pursuit of a policy decision.

A third perspective on the role of ethics is to see it as complementary to other forms of analysis. This view argues that ethical analysis adds distinctive content to the political-strategic assessment of nuclear policy, but that ethical analysis stands in need of other data in order to provide policy guidance. A complementary view of ethics and strategy affirms that ethics tells us something, but not enough to form policy judgments on either strategy or arms control. The Nye book and the bishops' pastoral letter are products of a complementary view of ethics and strategy. Both Bundy and Brzezinski implicitly use this model, but neither is clear about how ethical judgment is filtered through empirical data or how ethical choices might direct and define policy choices.

The future debate belongs to the complementary view of ethics and strategy. This model allows the paradoxical character of war and peace in the nuclear age to be analyzed prior to making ethical judgments, but it also holds firmly to the view that strategic and technological categories are incapable of defining the full range of human and political choices posed by nuclear weapons.

For three decades the political-strategic debate has been shaped by the concept of deterrence. One characteristic of the strategic debate in the 1980s, however, is the way in which the idea of deterrence has come under fire from several distinct perspectives. By the mideighties both the left and the right of the political spectrum were raising doubts about the viability of deterrence. Intrinsic to the critique of deterrence were moral arguments about either the "cost" (the economics of the arms race or the psychological costs of living with deterrence) or the "character" of deterrence (the targeting dilemmas).

Almost without warning, the idea that had been the organizing concept of the strategic debate in the 1960s and 1970s was itself the subject of debate. The future of this critique of deterrence is difficult to estimate. It is clearly easier to criticize deterrence than it is to replace it. Neither the Freeze, nor very deep cuts in weapons, nor the defensive options seem at present to have the capacity to dispel the hold of deterrence on our future. But the strategic literature and the speeches of statespersons as well as the fears and hopes of a newly engaged public all seem dissatisfied with a notion that there is nothing beyond deterrence.

When Nye tries to look at the long-term trend of reducing reliance on nuclear weapons, he distinguishes a political route and a technological route. The first is a road of managing the nuclear reality with a mix of arms control, evolution of political relationships, and careful strategic planning. The second is symbolized by the hopes of the advocates of the defensive option. My sense is that the future debate about ethics and strategy will have at least three lines of argument. Both prospects cited by Nye will be with us. The political-strategic road—how much arms control, what kind, which forces to deploy, what strategic doctrine to hold—will be a continuation of the discussion of the 1960s and 1970s, but not simply a linear extension of the past. Changes in the technology of nuclear forces, changes in public expectations, and changes in the way deterrence is viewed will all reshape this old argument.

The defensive option is now on the table, and some of its advocates press its moral superiority as its principal asset. I am unpersuaded by the argument, but it must be addressed. The complementary conception of ethics and strategy will be very useful here, for abstract moral claims of superiority must be tested against technological feasibility, strategic stability, and economic trade-offs which would have to be made in pursuit of a defensive future.

A third road for the debate will be the persistence of the Stein-Kenny position, particularly in the popular nuclear debate. The absence of this position among the strategists reviewed in this paper is understandable, but the position will not disappear.

In all three paths for the future the need for ethical analysis, argument, and advocacy is very evident. It will constitute a third stage of a discussion that took one form from 1960 to 1980 and another in the 1980s. The future will rely on both of these earlier moments but may not replicate either of them.

Notes

1. For an interpretation of some of these changes, see R. Tucker, *The Nuclear Debate: Deterrence and the Lapse of Faith* (New York: Holmes and Meier, 1985).

2. For a synthetic statement of this tradition, see R. B. Potter, *The Moral Logic of War* (Philadelphia: United Presbyterian Church, n.d.); J. F. Childress, "Just-War Theories," *Theological Studies* 39 (1978): 427–45.

3. Paul Ramsey, *The Just War: Force and Political Responsibility* (New York: Scribner's, 1968); and William V. O'Brien, "Just War Doctrine in a Nuclear Context," *Theological Studies* 44 (1983): 191–220.

4. Walter Stein, ed., *Nuclear Weapons and the Christian Conscience* (London: Merlin Press, 1961); and Anthony Kenny, *The Logic of Deterrence* (Chicago: University of Chicago Press, 1985).

5. Joseph S. Nye, Jr., *Nuclear Ethics* (New York: Free Press, 1986), 54.

6. Michael Walzer, *Just and Unjust Wars: A Moral Argument with Historical Illustrations* (New York: Basic Books, 1977), 270.

7. Ibid., 282.

8. Ibid., 254.

9. Ibid., 274.

10. National Conference of Catholic Bishops, *The Challenge of Peace: God's Promise and Our Response* (Washington, D.C.: United States Catholic Conference, 1983), 46–50.

11. Ibid., 58.

12. Ibid., 59–60.

13. Albert Wohlstetter, "Bishops, Statesmen and Other Strategists on the Bombing of Innocents," *Commentary* (June 1983), 15–35.

14. Ibid., 19.

15. Ibid., 22.

16. Ibid., 19.

17. McGeorge Bundy, "To Cap the Volcano," *Foreign Affairs* 48 (1969): 1–20.

18. McGeorge Bundy et al., "Nuclear Weapons and the Atlantic Alliance," *Foreign Affairs* 60 (1982): 753–68.

19. McGeorge Bundy, "The Bishops and the Bomb," *New York Review of Books* (June 16, 1983), 6.

20. Ibid., 3.

21. Ibid., 4.

22. Bundy, "Volcano," 17.

23. McGeorge Bundy, "Political Leadership and Nuclear Deterrence: Some Claims for the Utility of Truth," Remarks at the University of San Francisco (unpublished text), 8.

24. Ibid., 10.

25. Ibid., 10–15.

26. Nye, *Nuclear Ethics,* 52.

27. Ibid., 99ff.

28. Ibid., 56.

29. Zbigniew Brzezinski, "The Strategic Implications of Thou Shalt Not Kill," *America* (May 31, 1986), 445–49.

30. Ibid., 447.

31. Ibid., 448.

32. Keith B. Payne and Colin S. Gray, "Nuclear Policy and the Defensive Transition," *Foreign Affairs* 62 (1984): 820–42.

33. Donald Brennan, "The Case for Missile Defense," *Foreign Affairs* 48 (1969): 443ff.

34. Paul Nitze, *The Recovery of Ethics* (New York: CRIA, 1958).

II · RELIGIOUS STUDIES

**The Problematic
of Deterrence**

2 • The Morality of Nuclear Deterrence: Obstacles on the Road to Coherence

RICHARD B. MILLER

Over the past four decades, perhaps no ethical issue has stirred more emotional fervor and intellectual caution than nuclear deterrence, forcing ethicists to walk precipitously in the region between moral principle and political necessity in a world of vastly complex international relations. Moreover, with plans underway in public policy to enhance deterrence, especially by the Strategic Defense Initiative Organization,[1] questions surrounding the morality of deterrence assume new gravity: What are the bases for, and the limits of, deterrent threats? What is the logical and moral structure of deterrent intentions? What is the relation between the morality of using nuclear weapons and the morality of deterrence? To what extent can the facts of history be used to commend or critique deterrence?

Efforts to answer these questions take several forms, employ different methods, and invoke a variety of moral principles. Within this variety, however, four arguments presently constitute the conventional wisdom about nuclear deterrence, providing cautious and attractive justifications for the continuation of deterrent threats: the success thesis, the just-war thesis, the argument from "supreme emergency," and the exceptionalist thesis. The attraction of the success thesis lies in its appeal to the beneficial consequences of nuclear deterrence, namely, the prevention of nuclear war during the past forty years. The just-war thesis draws upon a well-known body of ethical wisdom to assess deterrence, appealing to what James Turner Johnson calls the "consensual tradition of Western culture" about the morality of war and peace.[2] The argument from supreme emergency focuses on the intractable problems posed by nuclear technology, leaving room for the limit situation of survival where it may be necessary to override traditional canons of morality. And the exceptionalist thesis grants philosophical validity to the intuition, especially attractive to the defenders of democracy against antidemocratic regimes, that one must assess the relative morality of opposing polities during times of conflict.

Yet despite these apparent attractions, this conventional wisdom about nuclear deterrence is gravely and dramatically ill-conceived. In this essay I will argue, in critical dialogue with representatives of the four arguments mentioned above, that the claims on behalf of deterrence are variously infected by inconsistencies, disanalogies, historical inaccuracies, practical difficulties, and logical fallacies. These obstacles to coherent reasoning exist at a variety of levels in moral and political discourse about nuclear policies, yet they remain hidden in the current debate about the justification and continuation of deterrent threats. As the debate goes forward, it is imperative to take stock of these problems facing deterrence, to uncover the errors concealed within the conventional wisdom, and to face soberly and critically the problems that beset a coherent and moral deterrent strategy.

The Success Thesis

Doubtless one of the most frequent claims found within the conventional wisdom is the apparent truth of deterrent success. Nuclear deterrence, it is held, has prevented a major conflict between the superpowers over the past four decades, and this success provides sufficient justification for the continued possession and improvement of the nuclear arsenal. The argument is, in essence, consequentialist: the positive benefit of nuclear deterrence—the fact that nuclear deterrence has worked—justifies the means necessary to render credible the threat of nuclear war in some form. As Caspar Weinberger remarks:

> [The policy of the United States] to prevent war since the age of nuclear weapons has been one of deterrence. . . . The idea on which this is based is quite simple: it is to make the cost of starting a nuclear war much higher than any possible benefit to an aggressor. This policy has been approved, through the political processes of the democratic nations it protects, since at least 1950. Most important, it works. It has worked in the face of major international tensions involving the great powers, and it has worked in the face of war itself.[3]

Assurances that deterrence has worked are legion in the scholarly debate. As Richard Wasserstrom observes in a recent double-issue of *Ethics* devoted to the subject of nuclear deterrence, "Our ideas about nuclear deterrence are all fixed within a context in which successful and effective threats are in one way or the other unreflectively presupposed."[4] Yet within the conventional wisdom the presupposition of success is more explicit than unreflective. Among noted historians, for example, William O'Brien states emphatically, "MAD [mutual assured destruction] . . . has in fact deterred superpower confrontations and nuclear war itself."[5] James Turner Johnson similarly asserts, "Thus far nuclear deterrence has been remarkably effective—ironically, a much better barrier to war than the Kellogg-Briand Treaty of 1927, the 'agreement to abolish war,' whose effect endured with manifest fragility for only a decade."[6] Indeed, the success thesis has been so much a part of accepted dogma within strategic circles that, as Solly Zuckerman states, "if a presumed intention of the USSR which was, or is, contrary to the West's political interests does not materialise, we conclude that it did not do so because the USSR feared a nuclear onslaught."[7] Among political essayists, Leon Wieseltier comes close to doubting the merits of the success thesis, but its irresistibility proves too much for him. Wieseltier remarks:

> Deterrence is often said to have "worked," and if anything has "worked," it has; but we cannot be sure. . . . To be a little more precise, deterrence is a proposition that may be known to be false, but not to be true. When it fails, we will know that it is false, or a few of us will. Until then we will persist in believing that it is true, and not entirely without reason. Deterrence is probably more than a necessary fiction and probably less than a law of history.[8]

Within religious ethics the success thesis has likewise made its mark. According to Robert McKim's careful analysis of the subtle shifts in the U.S. Catholic bishops' treatment of deterrence in the last three versions of their pastoral letter, the bishops were initially skeptical of the success thesis, "but never *so* skeptical that they are prepared to dismiss it."[9] The fact that the bishops grew progressively more reluctant to condemn nuclear deterrence, McKim argues, suggests that the success thesis became increasingly more attractive as they refined their argument. Reference to the success thesis is even more promiment, as we shall see, in David Hollenbach's attempt to provide guidelines for nuclear deterrence and future nuclear strategy.[10] Even the Methodist bishops, who condemn nuclear deterrence unequivocally, provide a muted acknowledgment of the success thesis when they say, "Whatever the objective truth about the effects of deterrence, faith in the doctrine will not die quickly."[11]

Despite its widespread popularity, the argument for success rests on an improper form of inductive reasoning. In the grammar of informal logic, to argue that the absence of war proves the success of deterrence is to embrace the *post hoc ergo propter hoc* fallacy. The success of nuclear deterrence is assumed to be true because certain facts exist, facts that would have to exist if the induction were to be true. Although much respectable inductive reasoning may involve *post hoc* argumentation, as J. L. Mackie instructively argues, the problem with the success thesis is that a simple concurrence of the threat of nuclear war and the lack of nuclear war is insufficient to establish a causal relation between them.[12] As is typical of fallacious *post hoc* arguments, the success thesis fails to eliminate rival hypotheses for the nonoccurrence of nuclear war, e.g., the absence of any strong motive of aggression on the part of the Soviets.[13]

One attempt to salvage the success thesis against the criticism of *post hoc* reasoning is to challenge this rival hypothesis by taking recourse to specific historical data, e.g., the Cuban missile crisis of 1962. In that instance the Soviets yielded to U.S. superiority and bellicose threats, and lacking such threats the United States would have been unable to deter undesirable Soviet behavior. Here, then, a positive correlation between deterrent threats and the absence of war seems relatively strong, lending credence to Weinberger's claim, "It has worked in the face of international tensions involving the great powers, and it has worked in the face of war itself."

Unfortunately, however, this use of history conceals at least one problem that proponents of the success thesis have failed to address. The problem can be stated rhetorically: If deterrence and nuclear strength are so effective, then what allowed the Soviets to act in the first place? The Cuban missile crisis is a case in which deterrence almost failed to prevent the outbreak of war, and certainly failed to deter the Soviets from taking initial steps of an adventurist sort. And, more importantly, such success presupposes a *deterioration* of nuclear deterrence as a prior condition of championing deterrent effectiveness. For, without this prior erosion of deterrence—the event of "the crisis"—there would be no context for citing the deterrent effectiveness of nuclear threats. The success thesis lacks the resources to account for this prior deterioration, even though it relies upon the context of crisis, in this case, for its intelligibility.

The use of history to support the success thesis is further complicated by the problem of predictability. Even if it were logically plausible to assert the success thesis, the *past* success of nuclear deterrence provides no guarantee of its *future* effectiveness. In the words of Sissela Bok, to conclude that nuclear weapons will not be used in the foreseeable future, based on the evidence of past nonuse, "requires a vast leap of inductive faith."[14] And, if the deterioration of nuclear deterrence serves as a prelude to at least some forms of deterrent success, then we clearly have more to fear than the success thesis would lead us to believe, for there is no necessary reason to think that future crises would be followed by successful deterrent threats.

A final problem with the success thesis emerges when one considers its implications for the use of nuclear weapons in the event of unsuccessful deterrence, that is, if deterrence fails. According to the success thesis, the possession of nuclear weapons is justified according to beneficial outcomes, namely, the prevention of nuclear war. It is also characteristic of representatives of the success thesis to insist that deterrence can be successful only if deterrent threats are backed by strategies to use nuclear weapons in some fashion.[15] Yet the implications of the success thesis are incoherent with strategies for use, because success presupposes that the use that is planned should never occur. As Wasserstrom remarks, "If using nuclear weapons, should deterrence fail, is required in order to promote successful deterrence, the two contexts of successful and unsuccessful deterrence are introduced within the same overall account, but only incoherently so."[16] For, once deterrence fails, the raison d'être for nuclear weapons (prevention of use) evanesces. Thus, using nuclear weapons would make little sense; indeed, such use would contradict the reason invoked to justify their existence in the first place.

Those who wish to follow the success thesis, then, are left with at least four obstacles on their road to coherence. First, if the beneficial consequences (prevention of use) justify the possession of nuclear weapons, then it would hardly make sense, in order to promote successful deterrence, to plan genuinely to use them, because such plans must presuppose a context in which nuclear deterrence has already failed. Indeed, using such weapons would subvert the very rationale for justifying their existence (again: nonuse). Second, efforts to cite prior specific instances of successful deterrence entail a prior erosion of deterrence to establish the context necessary for championing deterrent effectiveness. Moreover, such past successes, whatever sense can be made of them, furnish no guarantee of future deterrent effectiveness. Finally, these difficulties emerge only if one opts to ignore the most tenacious obstacle, namely, that appeals to success entail the fallacy of *post hoc ergo propter hoc* reasoning.

The Just-War Thesis

Representatives of the just-war thesis begin their arguments with a moral assessment of the use of nuclear weapons as a first step in their evaluations of nuclear deterrence. The general premise, in contrast to versions of the success thesis, is not that using nuclear weapons, should deterrence fail, is required to promote successful deterrence. Rather, the premise is that, if deterrence fails, the response to aggression should conform to the requirements of a just war. Thus, it is necessary to determine the moral limits of a nuclear war as a condition for a morally acceptable nuclear strategy. By making reference to the requirements of justice rather than effectiveness, moreover, representatives of the just-war thesis are not necessarily thwarted by the problem of *post hoc* reasoning in their moral permission of deterrent threats.

One of the most celebrated recent efforts to consider nuclear deterrence within the strictures of the just-war tradition is found in the pastoral letter of the U.S. Catholic bishops. The bishops begin their discussion of nuclear war and deterrence by affirming a fundamental tenet of the just-war tradition, namely, the imperative that war must be limited to discriminate and proportionate methods. Turning to the details of U.S. nuclear strategy, they identify three possible contingencies in which nuclear weapons might be used: countercity targeting, first-strike counterforce targeting, and second-strike counterforce targeting.

The gist of their analysis of the morality of using nuclear weapons is to apply the just-war tenets of discrimination and proportionality to these prospective uses, leading them to three conclusions. First, countercity strikes are immoral, contrary to the strict requirements of discrimination (noncombatant immunity). Moreover, and second, the use of counterforce nuclear weapons in a first strike stands outside the compass of just-war restraints, given the fact that counterforce nuclear war is likely to escalate beyond the control of its engineers. Even if the United States could cross the threshold from conventional to nuclear war according to discriminate methods, the bishops aver, the likelihood of escalation is such that the foreseen, unintended harms would far outweigh the putative values that are defended, contrary to the principle of proportionality. Drawing on the testimony of former public officials, the bishops aver, "The consequences involved in this problem lead us to conclude that the danger of escalation is so great that it would be morally unjustifiable to initiate nuclear war in any form. The danger is rooted not only in the technology of our weapons but also in the weakness and sinfulness of human communities. We find the moral responsibility of beginning nuclear war not justified by rational political objectives."[17] Third, about the morality of using nuclear weapons for second-strike counterforce purposes (that is, in response to the first use of nuclear weapons by an opponent), the bishops proceed cautiously. Despite the many statements in the document suggesting an endorsement of nuclear pacifism, they do *not* close the door on all uses of nuclear weapons. Choosing not to adjudicate the technical debate about the real possibility of fighting a limited nuclear war, the bishops instead pose a series of questions "which challenge the real meaning of 'limited.' " Would leaders have sufficient information about what is happening? Would precise decisions be possible? Could computer errors be avoided? "Unless these questions can be answered satisfactorily," they remark, "we will continue to be highly skeptical about the real meaning of 'limited.' " Backing off from a categorical judgment, the bishops instead place the burden of proof "on those who assert that meaningful limitation is possible."[18]

That the bishops leave open the possibility of second-strike counterforce is, as I shall show below, an incoherent position given their arguments against first-strike counterforce nuclear warfare. Their position does have the merit, however, of seeming to avoid the position of nuclear bluffing. For, with the door left slightly open to some form of nuclear warfare, it remains possible to endorse some forms of deterrence that can be backed with some credible, and morally acceptable, uses of nuclear weapons.

When turning directly to the morality of nuclear deterrence, the bishops structure their position according to the moral equivalence of action and intention. As they state in the summary, "No *use* of nuclear weapons which would violate the principles of discrimination or proportionality may be *intended* in a strategy of deterrence. The moral demands of Catholic teaching require resolute willingness not to intend or do moral evil even to save our own lives or the lives of those we love."[19] In keeping with their discussion of using nuclear weapons, then, the bishops are logically bound by this axiom of moral equivalence to proscribe countercity targeting or initiating a counterforce nuclear war as integral to a policy of nuclear deterrence, since their prior discussion of nuclear war according to just-war criteria concluded with such proscriptions. And, at least to some extent, this is how they argue. Concerning countercity targeting, the bishops maintain that "it is not morally acceptable to intend to kill the innocent as part of a strategy of deterring nuclear war." Strategies of massive retaliation are thus condemned, however much they might contribute to the prevention of nuclear war. About counterforce targeting, the bishops repeat their skepticism about the tenability of fighting and winning a nuclear war, noting the destabilizing effect of counterforce targeting on deterrent relations between the superpowers. They then conclude their analysis of deterrence by providing a "strictly conditioned moral acceptance" of nuclear deterrence, adding, "We cannot consider it adequate as a long-term basis for peace."[20]

The bishops articulate three conditions for accepting nuclear deterrence. They are

1. If nuclear deterrence exists only to prevent the *use* of nuclear weapons by others, then proposals to go beyond this to planning for prolonged periods of repeated nuclear strikes and counterstrikes, or "prevailing" in nuclear war, are not acceptable. They encourage notions that nuclear war can be engaged in with tolerable human and moral consequences. Rather, we must continually say "no" to the idea of nuclear war.
2. If nuclear deterrence is our goal, "sufficiency" to deter is an adequate strategy; the quest for nuclear superiority must be rejected.
3. Nuclear deterrence should be used as a step on the way toward disarmament. Each proposed addition to our strategic system or change in strategic doctrine must be assessed precisely in light of whether it will render steps toward "progressive disarmament" more or less likely.[21]

Barring these conditions, nuclear deterrence is unacceptable given the strictures of just-war tenets, and given the axiom of moral equivalence, in the bishops' reasoning.

The critical question that emerges for the bishops, however, is whether these three conditions are compatible with their judgments about fighting a nuclear war within the provenance of just-war tenets. That question must be answered negatively for each of the three conditions, leaving the bishops with an incoherent position on nuclear war and deterrence.

First, consider the bishops' discussion of the use of nuclear weapons in relation to the first condition they impose upon a morally acceptable nuclear deterrent. In their analysis of different uses of nuclear weapons within the compass of just-war criteria, the only form of nuclear war they do not completely condemn would be in response to an initial nuclear strike, that is, a counterstrike. And it would be highly imprudent to launch such a counterstrike unless one were cognizant of the very likely contingency that such a counterstrike would signal a willingness and ability to fight a limited nuclear war, creating a context for strikes and counterstrikes. The bishops *might* have in mind the hope that a counterstrike would generate sufficient fears on both sides to produce an immediate stalemate, without either side prevailing or continuing in battle. But as their proscription of initiating a nuclear war indicates, they hold to the notion that nuclear war cannot be kept limited, that stalemates are not conceivable, once the nuclear threshold has been crossed. Thus, their muted acceptance of the possibility of second-strike counterforce warfare is bound by their prior argument that limited war-fighting scenarios, and not stalemates, are virtually inevitable when resort to nuclear force occurs. However, if the bishops hold that using nuclear weapons in a second-strike counterforce manner commits one, or both, sides to a limited war-fighting situation, where the goal of prevailing is exigent, then their position on use and deterrence is incoherent, for the first condition for accepting deterrence is that it *cannot* be linked to a war-fighting strategy, that is, plans for "prevailing" in a nuclear war of "repeated nuclear strikes and counterstrikes." Unfortunately for the bishops, it is not possible to square the implications of their arguments about using nuclear weapons, and their muted acceptance of second-strike counterforce war, with this first condition imposed upon an acceptable nuclear deterrent.

One wonders, then, what sorts of uses would be acceptable to the bishops for a policy of nuclear deterrence, since the two other types of use—countercity and first-strike counterforce—have also been excluded according to their application of just-war criteria. The bishops' proscription of these two forms of nuclear warfare according to just-war criteria, together with their proscription of any nuclear war-fighting strategy as a condition for accepting nuclear deterrence, leave them with no real uses of nuclear weapons to support, or render credible, deterrent threats. Thus, without credible threats, the bishops have argued themselves into a position of nuclear bluffing, despite their apparent efforts to avoid such a conclusion.

Furthermore, the second condition—that " 'sufficiency' to deter is an adequate strategy; the quest for superiority must be rejected"—is incompatible with the material requirements for maintaining a second-strike counterforce capability. The reason here turns on the complex logic of deterrent strategy and incentives for arms competition in a counterforce world. To grasp this complex logic, assume for the moment two parties involved in a deterrent relation, A and B. Following the bishops' moral stance on the use of nuclear weapons, A adopts a deterrent strategy whereby it threatens to carry out retaliatory counterforce strikes against B's second-strike force, since, by definition, A's retaliatory strikes would be carried out after B launches an attack against A. Hence, A's retaliation must be targeted against B's second-strike force. The problem for the bishops is that the deployment of counterforce weapons by A generates incentives for B to develop its own counterforce capabilities to neutralize the threat to its own retaliatory forces posed by A. Without its retaliatory forces relatively secure, B's deterrent strength diminishes. And, once B develops weapons to neutralize A's threat, A must develop weapons to neutralize B's new weapons; otherwise, the threat posed by A's original counterforce arsenal has been nullified by B's newly developed weapons. The outcome is a cycle of competition whereby each gives the other incentives to build weapons, and where neither can feel secure absent a position of superiority.[22] But if, as the bishops argue, deterrence is unacceptable once it is linked to a "quest for superiority," then the material requirements for a second-strike counterforce arsenal cannot be satisfied.

The third condition posited by the bishops—that nuclear deterrence should be used as a step toward disarmament—is equally problematic. For, in a counterforce world fueled by arms competition, it is difficult to imagine how disarmament would be possible. In a competitive counterforce world the incentives are to build up one's reserve of nuclear weapons, not to disarm. How one can reconcile the bishops' call for progressive, bilateral disarmament with the material requirements of a second-strike counterforce strategy remains unclear.

Finally, as I have suggested above, it should be noted that *within* the bishops' analysis of counterforce nuclear war an inconsistency mars their discussion of first and second use. One possible use of nuclear weapons— to *initiate* a counterforce nuclear war—is deemed unacceptable according to just-war criteria. Yet when they turn to the possible use of nuclear weapons in a *second*-strike situation, they shift their ground. The earlier conclusion—that the dangers of escalation are so great as to render the initiation of nuclear war unjustifiable—now has a different conceptual force: doubts about limiting a nuclear war lead them to a grave skepticism, but not a categorical judgment. Yet if the danger of escalation rules out the first use of nuclear weapons, then the same danger should rule out *all* uses, since the danger of escalation is no less under the conditions of second use than under those of first use. Indeed, it is hard to see how the use of nuclear weapons in response to an initial strike is *itself* not a form of escalation. The trajectory of their argument against initiating a nuclear war, carried to its logical conclusion, ought to lead the bishops to the position of nuclear pacifism.[23]

A second representative of the just-war thesis, David Hollenbach, attempts to get beyond this last obstacle to the bishops' position about the morality of use by embracing the position of nuclear pacifism. Like the bishops, Hollenbach readily concludes that countercity strikes would be categorically immoral because they would be indiscriminate, violating the principle of noncombatant immunity. Yet Hollenbach goes beyond the bishops by concluding that, in all probability, *any* form of counterforce nuclear war would escalate beyond the control of its engineers, leading to disproportionate damage as a first step on the way to wanton mass destruction. Subsequent nuclear escalation, Hollenbach argues, would violate the *in bello* criteria of discrimination and proportionality, as well as the *ad bellum* criterion of reasonable hope of success.[24]

Given the axiom that immoral acts may never be morally intended, it would seem to follow from Hollenbach's line of reasoning that the intention to use nuclear weapons in either a counterforce or countercity strike is immoral. And, if the intention to use nuclear weapons is necessary to sustain a nuclear deterrent, then nuclear deterrence itself must be condemned. Yet in Hollenbach's mind it is necessary to separate our assessment of deterrence from the issue of use. Such a separation rests on understanding deterrent intentions as distinct, both logically and morally, from intentions to use nuclear weapons. The intention of nuclear deterrence is not the exercise of war, but the prevention of war. Assessments of nuclear deterrence, and the intentions of deterrence, must first come to terms with a fundamental paradox, namely, that "intention (nuclear war prevention) and action move in opposite directions."[25] Conceived in this way, deterrent intentions, in the words of Douglas MacLean, are "self-stultifying": they are structured so that, ideally, what is threatened will *not* be carried out.[26]

Commonplace discussions of the morality of nuclear deterrence often fail to develop the implications of this paradox. Such discussions often conclude that the morality of use is equivalent to the morality of deterrence. If this were the case, then Hollenbach's condemnation of use would necessarily yield a condemnation of nuclear deterrence. But if intentions to use and intentions to deter are logically separate, then the argument of moral equivalence does not hold. Thus, it becomes possible for Hollenbach to proscribe the use of nuclear weapons and still leave open the possibility for a morally acceptable deterrent, since this latter issue has now been wrenched free of considerations of use.

Yet Hollenbach does not wish to suggest that *all* deterrent intentions are equally tenable from either a moral or strategic point of view. His own effort to establish moral guidelines for deterrent intentions is couched in terms of revisionist proportionalism, a method of moral reasoning used in more liberal currents of contemporary Roman Catholic moral theology. Hollenbach remarks:

> One cannot determine what an agent intends to do without consider-ing the consequences which the agent foresees will follow from the contemplated action. If an agent chooses to perform an action whose good consequences are reasonably judged to be greater than are its evil consequences, this . . . school would judge that the intention is a morally upright one.[27]

Intention, within this framework, is determined not simply in terms of the objective, or goal, of one's choice, but also in terms of the foreseen consequences of one's choice. Determining what is actually intended in a deterrent threat should first include a reasonable prediction about what will result from making such a threat. Moral evaluations of deterrent in-tentions are thus contingent upon additional judgments about the pro-spective outcomes of any specific deterrent strategy. In Hollenbach's terms, the "moral judgment on the intention embodied in the deterrent policy is . . . inseparable from an evaluation of the reasonably predictable outcomes of diverse policy choices."[28]

Hollenbach is less interested in defending deterrence in principle than in providing criteria for assessing the moral wisdom of any shift in deter-rent policies. To this end he refines his considerations of "reasonably pre-dictable outcomes," specifying two goals toward which deterrent strate-gies should be ordered: (1) policies must make war less likely than policies presently in effect and (2) policy proposals must increase the possibility of arms reduction.[29] Any change in deterrence policy is acceptable to Hollenbach only if it can promise, in light of these criteria, to improve the status quo.

This argument on behalf of possessing nuclear weapons for purposes of deterrence, coupled with a condemnation of use, is an argument that is tantamount to nuclear bluffing. The difficulty here turns on the issue of credibility in public policy: no one will believe such threats if they are tied to a condemnation of use. Hollenbach acknowledges this difficulty, but he defends his argument for "threats without use" by taking recourse to the success thesis. We must note, Hollenbach states, "one single, historical fact: large numbers of nuclear weapons are already deployed and ready for use by both superpowers. Though incompatible on the level of ideas and logic, deterrence and non-use are concretely and existentially interlocked in our present world."[30] Thus, for Hollenbach, the problem of credibility for the "threat without use" is pertinent in the realm of abstract logic, but credibility becomes a nonproblem once we recognize the historical success of nuclear deterrence—the concrete interlocking of "deterrence and non-use."

One clear strength of Hollenbach's contribution to the debate about deterrence is that his criteria require us to think about the future direction of deterrent policy. The effect of his argument is to shift moral analysis from looking backward to looking ahead, moving us beyond moral judgments that lament the dawn of the nuclear age. Thus, he places the onus of responsibility on those who have inherited the task of managing nuclear policies but who were in no way directly involved in their creation.

Despite this strength, four distinct problems mar Hollenbach's challenging contribution to the debate about the morality of deterrence. First, there is a problem surrounding his reference to history to support his case for the credibility of a "threat without use" nuclear deterrent. Even if, as Hollenbach argues, "deterrence and non-use are concretely and existentially interlocked in our present world," this "interlocking" cannot be attributed historically to a policy of "threat without use." As Lawrence Freedman's magisterial study of the history of nuclear strategy indicates, deterrent strategy in the United States consistently has been premised on threats that have been backed by a readiness and willingness to use nuclear weapons under specified conditions.[31] And, according to Paul Bracken's more recent study, present command and control systems are now mechanized so that the release of nuclear weapons under the situation of attack would be virtually automatic.[32] As such, if we place nuclear strategy within its actual historical context, it becomes clear that deterrence must be "interlocked" to a policy of threats that are backed by a genuine readiness to use nuclear weapons, *not threats that are linked to a policy of nuclear pacifism.* History, then, cannot come to the aid of arguments for nuclear pacifism when they are criticized, in light of the requirements of deterrence, as incredible.

Second, the material requirements of Hollenbach's "threat without use" theory are morally unfeasible. By this I do not mean that his position is not credible, but that there are moral problems that surround making it credible *as an institution.* Even if it were possible to institutionalize a "threat without use" policy at the highest levels of military command, the consent to use nuclear weapons must be institutionalized in the *praxis* of lower-level officials who consent to carry out commands, or assume command, in a crisis. Unless one is willing to argue that *everyone* involved in the chain of command should know that nuclear weapons would *never* be used (hardly a credible policy), then one must grant that even a bluffing policy entails the cooperation to use nuclear weapons by lower-level individuals who would authorize, or who intend to carry out, the release of nuclear weapons.[33] Essential to such cooperation are human intentions that remain open to acts that Hollenbach has proscribed according to just-war criteria.

Third, Hollenbach's attention to the moral problems of unsuccessful deterrence, coupled with his reference to the success thesis to ward off the problems of incredibility, place him in a curious bind. If deterrence is successful, then the moral issues surrounding unsuccessful deterrence (i.e., whether any uses of nuclear weapons would be acceptable) are moot. Yet, if unsuccessful deterrence is a genuine problem, a real possibility calling for moral analysis aided by just-war criteria, then the success of deterrence cannot be a secure anchor for thinking about nuclear policies. And, if the success of deterrence is not secure, neither is the basis on which Hollenbach solves the problem of credibility as it pertains to his theory of "threat without use." To paraphrase Wasserstrom, if not using nuclear weapons, should deterrence fail, is required by just-war tenets, and if deterrence and nonuse are "concretely and existentially interlocked in our present world," the two contexts of unsuccessful and successful deterrence are introduced into the same overall account, but incoherently so.

Finally, it is not clear that Hollenbach's argument for "threats without use" can pass his own test for assessing the moral tenability of specific policy choices. If, as he maintains, the "moral judgment of the intention embodied in the deterrent policy is . . . inseparable from an evaluation of the reasonably predictable outcomes of diverse policy choices," then it remains unclear whether Hollenbach's position, *taken as a whole,* has been sufficiently established. For, given this definition of intention, it would seem necessary to show that proscribing the use of nuclear weapons and maintaining possession for deterrent purposes will yield, in all likelihood, a positive outcome. Unfortunately, his appeal to the success thesis to establish a positive outcome is logically and historically untenable, as I have argued above.

The Argument from the Supreme Emergency

A third attempt to justify nuclear deterrence, by Michael Walzer, begins with an assessment of nuclear war within the compass of just-war restraints, but emphasizes the qualitatively unique dangers of the nuclear era and the virtually intractable moral situation in which we find ourselves. The objective is to leave some room for the requirements of necessity, at least in extreme cases of unmitigated disaster.[34] Thus, the position is not entirely bound by the demands of justice, and the obstacles therein, characteristic of the just-war thesis.

Interestingly, Walzer's argument anticipates by several years the chief currents within the bishops' and Hollenbach's arguments. Like the bishops, Walzer begins by embracing the axiom of equivalence between intention and action. Yet, like Hollenbach, Walzer insists that no uses of nuclear weapons, under the ordinary circumstances of war, could pass the test of just-war criteria. In Walzer's terms, nuclear weapons "explode the theory of the just war." As the case of Hiroshima illustrates, nuclear destruction wreaks "indiscriminate slaughter, the killing of the innocent . . . on a massive scale."[35] Accordingly, if the use of nuclear weapons is murder, then the intention to use such weapons is a commitment to murder. Thus, Walzer notes, nuclear deterrence must be condemned insofar as it relies on such an intention.

Yet having arrived at this judgment, Walzer proceeds to embrace the arguments of those who are sympathetic to nuclear deterrence. Generally these arguments make some reference to the success thesis, pointing to the putative beneficial consequences of nuclear deterrence. Historically, nuclear deterrence has been fashioned under the banner "Better dead than Red," and has furnished the best safeguard against the twofold danger of nuclear blackmail and nuclear destruction.[36]

Moreover, Walzer notes, the dangers surrounding nuclear war are qualitatively different from the dangers of conventional war. Thus, it is simplistic to draw upon moral criteria that derive from conventional, rather than nuclear, contexts. Moral analysis must adjust its sights to the different stakes in the nuclear age:

> The case is very different from that which arises commonly in war, where *our* adherence to the war convention puts us, or would put us, at a disadvantage vis-à-vis *them*. For disadvantages of that sort are partial and relative; various countermeasures and compensating steps are always available. But in the nuclear case, the disadvantage is absolute. Against an enemy actually willing to use the bomb, self-defense is impossible, and it makes sense to say that the only compensating step is the (immoral) threat to respond in kind.[37]

Walzer draws on his notion of the supreme emergency to buttress his argument on behalf of compensating deterrent threats. Such an emergency, in Walzer's sense, "is defined by two criteria . . . : the first has to do with the imminence of the danger and the second with its nature." Under the circumstances of dire and imminent danger, when conventional methods of resistance are hopeless, "anything goes," that is, anything necessary to win. A supreme emergency allows one to override strict moral principle (e.g., noncombatant immunity) in the limit situation of survival, the situation in which "our history will be nullified and our future condemned unless I accept the burdens of criminality here and now."[38]

Supreme emergency is particularly relevant to nuclear issues, in Walzer's mind, because nuclear weapons now pose an imminent and irreversible danger to the international order. Indeed, Walzer claims that supreme emergency is now a "permanent condition" of international relations, where nuclear deterrence is the only available means for stabilizing relations in a world of sovereign states. Given the stakes involved in the nuclear age, nuclear deterrence should not be judged solely in terms of murderousness; instead, we must make some concessions to necessity. Thus, Walzer notes, nuclear deterrence may be the least evil strategy at our disposal: "We threaten evil in order not to do it, and the doing of it would be so terrible that the threat seems in comparison to be morally defensible.[39]

Walzer formulates a position, then, that is uniquely suited to deal with special problems in war, like those in which one is forced to confront an enemy who systematically violates moral codes. His theory of the supreme emergency, for example, allows for considerations of necessity against the perils of Nazism. With their "backs to the wall" against such an enemy, the Allies were on the edge of moral experience, proceeding along the precipice of desperation and disaster. And it is this kind of limit situation that constitutes our present condition. Like the early Allied bombing of German cities, Walzer suggests, nuclear deterrence is an act of necessity, placing us in the moral paradox where "we move uneasily beyond the limits of justice for the sake of justice (and of peace)."[40]

Unfortunately, however, Walzer equivocates about the meaning and ethical implications of a supreme emergency, leading him to a position that creates problems for moral reasoning. On the one hand, supreme emergency denotes a discrete, extraordinary event, one that requires unique moral decisions on the boundary of ordinary human experience. At such a precipice, we may violate the requirements of justice so that the conditions of justice might be restored. On the other hand, Walzer calls the supreme emergency a permanent condition in the nuclear age; it is not an extreme case on the edge of an otherwise ordinary set of conditions, but an extreme set of conditions now defining the context of international relations and the problems therein.

Coordinating the ethical implications of the first and second senses of supreme emergency generates two specific problems for Walzer's argument. First, if supreme emergency in the first sense establishes conditions for violating moral laws in the name of necessity, then what can we say about moral laws under conditions in which the supreme emergency is permanent? It appears that, for Walzer, nuclear deterrence can be justified because *anything* can be justified between the superpowers in the name of necessity now that the emergency has been construed in permanent terms. The effect of Walzer's argument is not to provide a principled justification for nuclear deterrence, but to define a set of conditions in which moral principles lose their force. And because the emergency is permanent, so is the eclipse of moral principle.

A second difficulty follows. The outcome of Walzer's position is to commit himself, and those who follow his lead, to a notion of superpower relations in which expectations of morality are now permanently effaced. One implication is that it is now impossible to hold others accountable to moral principles, since in the permanent condition of the supreme emergency, necessity and not moral principle is the law of the land. The effect of Walzer's argument leaves him in a difficult bind: it may be possible to justify one's own deterrent threats, but it is impossible to condemn as irrevocably evil the threats expressed by one's opponents.

Thus, for those who follow Walzer's lead, two stubborn obstacles remain. First, there appear to be no moral limits between the superpowers in the nuclear era, now that supreme emergency has become a permanent condition; second, and as a result of this first problem, Walzer is unable to discriminate morally between the necessities of one superpower polity and another in a supreme emergency.

The Exceptionalist Thesis

Arguing that Walzer's difficulties stem from his liberal political philosophy, Gerald Mara turns to classical sources to salvage the notion of supreme emergency from the problem of moral limits and the problem of discriminating between the necessities of different polities in a supreme emergency, permanently construed. Drawing from the political philosophy of Aristotle, Mara argues that the task of political order is to create virtuous citizens and to create an ethos that simultaneously mirrors and reinforces virtuous behavior. Accordingly, Mara notes, different political regimes can "be evaluated in terms of how well *their* particular values match the life that is most desirable for members of the human species."[41] It thus becomes possible to discriminate morally between regimes, and to criticize various regimes for failing to create the conditions for human well-being and moral action.

The effect of Mara's argument is to furnish grounds for distinguishing between different kinds of necessity in war, corresponding to the relative goodness of political regimes. Necessity, within this perspective, takes on varying moral force, depending on "the dominant community values that are in jeopardy."[42] There are notable differences between the morality of one regime and another, and such differences can make all the difference when it comes to justifying acts in the name of necessity. Mara notes:

A well-ordered, just society appeals to a different type of necessity in defense of *its* ultimate values than does a rapacious and tyrannical one. When evil regimes are placed (or place themselves) in situations where additional crimes are *truly* necessary to preserve their collective identities, they appeal to a kind of necessity that is nearly subhuman in nature. There is a difference between an appeal to necessity in the name of survival alone and an appeal in the name of survival and justice.[43]

Yet there are also resources within an Aristotelian perspective, Mara observes, to restrict a good regime's recourse to the rationale of necessity. Resort to necessity must be judged in terms of its effects on the quality of life within a regime: "Within Aristotle's perspective, means are not related to ends merely instrumentally. Rather, practical actions taken in pursuit of some good materially affect the actor's capacity to achieve or enjoy that good."[44] And, Mara notes, this truth about the dynamic relation between moral action and individual character pertains to the character, or ethos, of communities. Reference to necessity, over the long haul, will affect the character or ethos of a community, contributing to a cheapening of the value of life. This is especially the case with communities which commit themselves, as a strategy of deterrence, to threats of massively destructive acts; such threats will poison the character of life within the community making those threats. And if the goodness of a community is determined by the extent to which it conduces to virtue and eudaimonia among its citizens, then there are strong moral reasons to be critical of nuclear deterrence as one symptom of a permanent condition.

In essence, then, Mara seems to chart a way over the obstacles to Walzer's notion of the supreme emergency, without capitulating to the current regime of nuclear weapons: reference to the moral differences between opposing polities allows one to retain moral conventions in superpower relations, and allows one to distinguish relative differences between one version of emergency and another in times of conflict.

Nevertheless, Mara's attempt to salvage Walzer's theory is not without three grave difficulties, of which the first two are ethical and the third is historical. The first problem is that of exceptionalism within moral judgments about necessity and duress. Mara's position allows a nation, or an alliance, to make special claims for itself by referring to the superior morality of its own political order when juxtaposed to the relative evil of an opponent. Accordingly, in a time of duress, one party may commit acts that would be condemned if the opponent were to carry them out instead. The argument opens the door to a double standard in judgments about war and necessity, allowing one polity to exempt itself from the standards by which it judges another polity's wartime acts. And if the supreme emergency is a permanent condition, as Walzer maintains, it seems doubtful that there can be resources within Mara's position to curb the ongoing possibility of self-justifying abuse.

Second, Mara's position is problematic for most Christian ethicists insofar as it ascribes final or supreme value to human community, especially the nation-state. Christian ethicists, in general, would be averse to assigning ultimate value to the survival of the nation-state, given the fact that human communities are, at most, relative rather than absolute values.[45] Within the framework of Christian ethics it is more difficult to cite the moral goodness of the community as a warrant for overriding moral duties, like that of noncombatant immunity, unless one is willing to relate the survival of the nation-state, or an alliance of states, to divine purposes.[46]

Third, the gravest question for Mara is whether the modern nation-state bears sufficient similarity to the Aristotelian polis to justify his attempt to think about the modern situation along Aristotelian lines. As Alasdair MacIntyre has recently and trenchantly argued in his own attempt to retrieve Aristotelian ideas for post-Enlightenment philosophy, modern government owes more to the instrumental practices of post-Weberian rationalism than to Aristotle's idea of an authentic political and moral community. In "advanced societies," MacIntyre notes, "government does not express or represent the moral community of its citizens, but is instead a set of institutional arrangements for imposing a bureaucratized unity on a society which lacks genuine moral consensus." In contrast, the polis fosters an authentic sense of community and political representation, where patriotism is "founded primarily to a political and moral community and only secondarily to the government of that community."[47] Juxtaposed to MacIntyre's Aristotelian critique of the modern nation-state, Mara's position seems anachronistic, one which fails to distinguish the conditions for an authentic community from large, industrial, institutional societies.

Mara anticipates this criticism, arguing that " the hostility of modern society to virtuous practice—noted by MacIntyre, for example—appears to be a conclusion to be firmly established rather than preemptively stated," and that "it is as encouraging as it is intimidating to realize that adopting the classical perspective is a commitment to developing and asking certain questions rather than the process of applying principles that are foregone conclusions."[48] But Mara fails to suggest how modern society might attain the moral consensus, and the corresponding sense of patria and authentic political representation, that render intelligible Aristotle's notion of community. For, without these Aristotelian presuppositions, there would seem to be no basis for Mara to judge the relative ability of a community to foster virtuous practices and the realization of eudaimonia. MacIntyre's critique of modernity points to a grave disanalogy between the modern nation-states and the Aristotelian polis, a disanalogy which has philosophical, political, and sociological dimensions, and which undermines Mara's effort to salvage the supreme emergency along classical lines in the present age.

Conclusion

Each of the arguments cited above—the success thesis, the just-war thesis, the argument from supreme emergency, and the exceptionalist thesis—attempts to furnish, if not a moral rationale, at least a framework to salvage nuclear deterrence as a plausible moral institution. There is no doubt that a massive bureaucratic institution within the U.S. military has been fashioned out of deterrent policies, that individuals and groups have committed themselves to the maintenance and improvement of the nuclear arsenal, and that the institution is likely to continue—however complex the ethical debate may be. But if these four arguments provide a clue, then nuclear deterrence remains an institution, with a corresponding set of financial and practical commitments, that is manifestly bereft of a clear and consistent argument. For those of all stripes—pacifists and just-war theorists—it is clear that such a state of affairs affords little comfort. Thus, as the current debate about the morality of nuclear deterrence goes forward, it is timely that we take cognizance of the many obstacles along the way, logical and practical obstacles that we continue to overlook only at our collective peril.[49]

Notes

1. For a discussion of the Strategic Defense Initiative and its relation to nuclear deterrence, see United Methodist Council of Bishops, *In Defense of Creation: The Nuclear Crisis and a Just Peace* (Nashville, Tenn.: Graded Press, 1986), 49–52; James R. Schlesinger, "Rhetoric and Realities in the Star Wars Debate," in Steven E. Miller and Stephen Van Erva, eds., *The Star Wars Controversy, An International Security Reader* (Princeton: Princeton University Press, 1986), 15–24, esp. 17–18; and Joseph Nye, Jr., *Nuclear Ethics*

(New York: Free Press, 1986), 125. All of these sources note how the rationale for the Strategic Defense Initiative has shifted from "rendering nuclear weapons obsolete" (in order to move away from the immorality of deterrence) to *enhancing* deterrence. Obviously the shift in rationale entails a shift in the moral evaluation of deterrence.

2. James Turner Johnson, *Can Modern War Be Just?* (New Haven: Yale University Press, 1984), 1. See Johnson's study of the development of just-war ideas, *Just War Tradition and the Restraint of War: A Moral and Historical Inquiry* (Princeton: Princeton University Press, 1981).

3. Caspar Weinberger, "A Rational Approach to Nuclear Disarmament," in James Sterba, ed., *The Ethics of Nuclear War and Deterrence* (Belmont, Calif.: Wadsworth Books, 1985), 117.

4. Richard Wasserstrom, "War, Nuclear War, and Nuclear Deterrence: Some Conceptual and Moral Issues," *Ethics* 95 (April 1985): 435–40.

5. William V. O'Brien, *The Conduct of Just and Limited War* (New York: Praeger Publishers, 1981), 138.

6. Johnson, *Can Modern War Be Just?*, 103.

7. Solly Zuckerman, *Nuclear Illusion and Reality* (New York: Vintage Books, 1983), 48.

8. Leon Wieseltier, "The Great Nuclear Debate," *New Republic* (January 10 and 17, 1983), 35. Wieseltier subsequently published this extended essay as *Nuclear War, Nuclear Peace* (New York: H. Holt, 1983).

9. Robert McKim, "An Examination of Moral Argument against Nuclear Deterrence," *Journal of Religious Ethics* 13 (Fall 1985): 279–97, at 283–85.

10. David Hollenbach, S.J., *Nuclear Ethics: A Christian Moral Argument* (New York: Paulist Press, 1983), 83.

11. *In Defense of Creation*, 49.

12. *Encyclopedia of Philosophy*, 1st ed., s.v. "Fallacies," by J. L. Mackie. That this is an inductive fallacy, one which pertains to the relation of facts to themselves, means that it is also vulnerable to the charge that it issues in a falsehood. That is, the fallacy obscures other nonnuclear accounts for the absence of war (see note 13).

13. For a brief discussion of nonnuclear factors contributing to the absence of war, see McGeorge Bundy, "Existential Deterrence and Its Consequences," in Douglas MacLean, ed., *The Security Gamble: Deterrence Dilemmas in the Nuclear Age* (Totowa, N.J.: Rowman and Allanheld Publishers), 6–8.

14. Sissela Bok, "Distrust, Secrecy, and the Arms Race," *Ethics* 95 (April 1985): 716.

15. See, for example, Johnson, *Can Modern War Be Just?*, chs. 5, 6, and 8, and O'Brien, *Just and Limited War*, ch. 6. In more recent writings, O'Brien has placed tighter restraints on the use of nuclear force than he did in his previous writings. See William V. O'Brien, "The Failure of Deterrence and the Conduct of War," in William V. O'Brien and John Langan, S.J., eds., *The Nuclear Dilemma and the Just War Tradition* (Lexington, Mass.: Lexington Books, 1986), 153–97, at 158, 176.

16. Wasserstrom, "Nuclear Deterrence," 440; see also Jonathan Schell, *The Fate of the Earth* (New York: Alfred A. Knopf, 1982), 197. The problem of introducing notions of successful and unsuccessful deterrence into the same overall account is particularly acute for O'Brien's argument. His entire argument on behalf of a counterforce war-fighting strategy as essential to a credible deterrent begins with the assumption "that the nuclear deterrent has failed, aggression has occurred, and a nuclear response of some kind is under consideration." See O'Brien, *Just and Limited War*, 129, and, more recently, "The Failure of Deterrence," 153, 156.

17. National Conference of Catholic Bishops, *The Challenge of Peace: God's Promise and Our Response* (Washington, D.C.: United States Catholic Conference, 1983), 48.

18. *The Challenge of Peace*, 49–50. It should be noted, moreover, that the bishops are considering "the *real* as opposed to the *theoretical* possibility of a 'limited nuclear exchange' " (emphasis theirs).

19. Ibid., iii–iv.

20. Ibid., 58.

21. Ibid., 59.

22. For a discussion of the present counterforce and retaliatory capabilities in the U.S. arsenal, see Barry R. Posen and Stephen Van Erva, "Defense Policy and the Reagan Administration: Departure from Containment," *International Security* 8 (Summer 1983): 3–45.

23. For a similar view of the bishops' argument on the issue of use, see William E. Murnion, "The American Catholic Bishops' Peace Pastoral: A Critique of Its Logic," *Horizons* (Spring 1986), 79–80. Moreover, this problem of reconciling the proscription of a nuclear first strike with the permission of second-strike counterforce warfare also plagues the argument for a "no first use" policy made by four former U.S. officials. See McGeorge Bundy, George F. Kennan, Robert McNamara, and Gerard Smith, "Nuclear Weapons and the Atlantic Alliance," *Foreign Affairs* 60 (Spring 1982): 753–68.

24. Hollenbach, *Nuclear Ethics*, 47–62.

25. Ibid., 65.

26. MacLean, Introduction to *The Security Gamble*, xvii.

27. Hollenbach, *Nuclear Ethics*, 57.

28. Ibid., 74.

29. Ibid., 75.

30. Ibid., 83.

31. Lawrence Freedman, *The Evolution of Nuclear Strategy* (New York: St. Martin's Press, 1983), esp. chs. 4–9, 14–16, 25. See also Desmond Ball, "U.S. Strategic Forces: How Would They Be Used?" *International Security* 7 (Winter 1982–83): 31–60, esp. 33–40.

32. Paul Bracken, *The Command and Control of Nuclear Forces* (New Haven: Yale University Press, 1983), 179–237.

33. For a similar point, see Anthony Kenny, *The Logic of Deterrence* (Chicago: University of Chicago Press, 1985), 50, 53–54.

34. Michael Walzer, *Just and Unjust Wars: A Moral Argument with Historical Illustrations* (New York: Basic Books, 1977), 269–83. For a retrieval of the supreme emergency as analogous with Vitoria's application of just-war ideas, see Johnson, *Can Modern War Be Just?*, 185–90. See also the recent discussions of Walzer's notion of the supreme emergency by Gerald Mara (to be discussed below), Hollenbach, and O'Brien in O'Brien and Langan, *The Nuclear Dilemma*, 15–18, 49–64, 227–28.

35. Walzer, *Just and Unjust Wars*, 272.

36. Ibid., 273.

37. Ibid., 273–74.

38. Ibid., 252, 260.

39. Ibid., 274.

40. Ibid., 253, 282.

41. Gerald M. Mara, "Justice, War, and Politics: The Problem of Supreme Emergency," in O'Brien and Langan, *The Nuclear Dilemma*, 49–78.

42. Ibid., 70.

43. Ibid., 67.

44. Ibid.

45. See, for example, *The Challenge of Peace*, 74, where the "real but relative" value

of national sovereignty is affirmed. The relativity of national sovereignty precludes reference to national survival as an ultimate value or principle, even within the present international order.

46. One such example is Jerram Barrs, *Who Are the Peacemakers: The Christian Case for Nuclear Deterrence,* with an introduction by Francis Schaeffer (Westchester, Ill.: Crossway Books, 1983).

47. Alasdair MacIntyre, *After Virtue: A Study in Moral Theory* (Notre Dame, Ind.: University of Notre Dame Press, 1981), 236–37.

48. Mara, "Justice, War, and Politics," 71.

49. I would like to thank members of the Multidisciplinary Seminar, "The Experience of War," at Indiana University; Mary Jo Weaver; and the anonymous readers for *Horizons* for their useful criticisms of earlier drafts of this essay.

3 • Ethics in Distress: Can There Be Just Wars in the Nuclear Age?

DAVID HOLLENBACH, S.J.

In the recent literature on the ethics of war, a vocabulary has come increasingly into use that provides a point of entry into the current debate on justice and war in the nuclear age. If an index of key words in the recent ecclesiastical pronouncements and scholarly analyses of the ethics of warfare were available, the references under *crisis, emergency, tension,* and *distress* would direct one to some of the most challenging passages of these documents. Every sane person knows, of course, that the employment of a significant number of the nuclear weapons deployed today would be a crisis or emergency for humanity of extreme magnitude. My interest in this vocabulary, however, has a different and less apocalyptic focus. These words are used in contexts that suggest not only that the realities of contemporary nuclear strategy may be in conflict with the traditions of Western and Christian ethical thought, but also that we may be faced with policy choices that are simply not analyzable in terms of traditional moral categories. If this is the case, we would be confronted not only with the possible crisis of an actual nuclear war, but also with a crisis of moral reason itself. Ethics would itself be in distress. It is my intention in this chapter to examine the reasons that have led to the emergence of this language of distress, to ask whether these reasons really imply a crisis of moral reason, and to explore what can be done about this situation.

The Situation of Distress

It will be useful to begin by pointing out some of the passages I have in mind in the recent literature. They occur principally in the context of the discussion of the morality of nuclear deterrence, especially those forms of deterrence that threaten to attack urban populations. For example, the Roman Catholic bishops of France, in their pastoral letter of November 8,

1983, were willing to justify the threat to use the French *force de frappe* as a means of deterring both nuclear blackmail and actual Warsaw Pact aggression against France. They argued that a smaller power like France can achieve a "deterrence of the strong by the weak" through possession and threat to use weapons capable of inflicting "intolerable damage upon a much more powerful aggressor." The bishops acknowledge that the French strategy involves a threat to attack cities, and point out that such countercity attacks were "condemned, clearly and without appeal" by the Second Vatican Council. They then note that "threat is not use" and reply to the question of whether the immorality of use makes the threat immoral with a rather vague response: "That is not evident." They are pressed to this conclusion by what they call "a logic of distress." Indeed, they state that their conclusion embodies an "ethic of distress."[1] Their exact meaning is not spelled out, but it does seem to imply the existence of an inner moral tension in their conclusion. It may even contain a moral contradiction that is made tolerable only by the present lack of more acceptable alternatives and that must be overcome as soon as possible. A "situation of distress" makes bedfellows of moral purpose and the threat to do the immoral.

The Catholic bishops of West Germany have been led to a similar sort of conclusion. They characterize their temporary tolerance of a threat to do that which they judge to be immoral as acceptance of an "emergency system" (*Notordnung*) that is needed until we can find an alternative. The realities of the conflict between East and West press them to adopt an "emergency set of ethics" (*Notstandethik*).[2] The emergency to which they refer is the "immense tension" at the heart of nuclear strategy. This cord of tension has two strands.

The first concerns the *goals* of policy. Nuclear strategy seeks to defend against "injustice, oppression and totalitarian extortion." It also seeks to prevent the "horror" that war, conventional or nuclear, between the superpowers would bring.[3] These twin goals of the protection of justice and the prevention of war cannot be considered a single unified objective. Indeed, a single-minded pursuit of one of them can threaten the other. The relation between the dual ends of justice and peace has been analyzed extensively through the history of the just-war tradition. The German bishops suggest, however, that the nuclear weapons deployed on both sides of the East-West divide have raised it to a level that deserves to be called an emergency.

The second strand of policy concerns the *means* employed in nuclear strategy. Here the tension is between the direction in which these means carry us and the ends that have pressed us to develop these means. Nuclear force structures and targeting doctrines are designed to protect justice and secure peace. There is a serious danger, however, that these means could subvert one or both of the goals they seek to secure. In fact, present nuclear strategies are based on means that, if used, would violate both just-war norms and fundamental human rights. The emergency ethic of which the German bishops speak is based on an acknowledgment that such a subversion of the ends of strategy by its means is a distinct possibility in the nuclear age. Their toleration of the legitimacy of these means, despite the risks entailed, is anguished: "By virtue of this decision we are choosing from among various evils the one which, as far as it is humanly possible to tell, appears as the smallest."[4] Their dissatisfaction with this "emergency ethic" is evident in their repeated plea that some better arrangement must be created. Although they express a true Christian trust that "with God all things are possible," nevertheless, their optimism on the political level is not great:

> Those who rely on this will never be able to accept the existing conditions (cf. Mk 9:23). Such people are summoned to hope against hope (cf. Rom 4:18). . . . We know from the gospel that this emergency situation is not the final word in worldly wisdom, for God's wisdom is not our wisdom.[5]

Here the German bishops come close to saying that efforts to bring nuclear strategy under the direction of moral reason have not succeeded and that our only recourse is to a religious trust that God will extract us from this situation of distress. This response, though understandable, is a curious one, for although Roman Catholic theology has a very strong doctrine of divine providence, it has never viewed God's providence and human responsibility as antithetical to each other. As Thomas Aquinas stated, human beings are rational beings and, as such, "participate in providence by their own providing for themselves and others."[6] The problem that leads the German bishops to this transmoral religious cri de coeur is that it is far from clear just how we are to provide for ourselves and others under the nuclear shadow.

Michael Walzer has stated the problem in the most explicit and challenging terms. Walzer, no utilitarian, therefore strongly rejects most tendencies to collapse the moral criteria for the justice of warfare into the single norm of proportionality. He sees efforts to determine the morality of warfare solely on the basis of a comparative weighing of goods and evils as stumbling on the difficulty of weighing different kinds of incommensurable values against each other. Further, the norm of proportionality is a "weak constraint," lacking the "creative power"[7] to set definite limits on war. It must therefore be supplemented, as the just-war tradition has long known, by a firm principle of noncombatant immunity from direct attack.

Walzer, however, is prepared to suspend this noncombatant immunity constraint in the situation he calls "supreme emergency." The phrase, borrowed from Churchill, refers to military-political circumstances where the fundamental values of civilization are in imminent danger of being destroyed or overthrown.[8] Walzer appealed to this line of reasoning to justify the initial instances of British saturation bombing of German cities during World War II. In his view, there was simply no alternative way to resist the massive evil being perpetrated by the Nazi regime. Walzer argued that this justification ceased as soon as other means for defending the fundamental values of civilization became available.

The status of the moral justification Walzer offers for these indiscriminate area bombings, however, remains ambiguous. On the one hand, he declares them to be legitimate. On the other hand, he states that those who ordered and carried out the bombings must be willing to "accept the burdens of criminality here and now." This criminality is not only a violation of a legal code but also a transgression of moral norms:

> The deliberate killing of the innocent is murder. Sometimes, in conditions of extremity (which I have tried to define and delimit) commanders must commit murder or they must order others to commit it. And then they are murderers, though in a good cause.[9]

Walzer is fully aware that this conclusion is self-contradictory. Although not all killing is immoral according to just-war tradition, all murder surely is. Murder, by definition, is unjustified killing. To declare it morally legitimate is to make a nonsensical statement: this act is both justified and unjustified at the same time. It is to state, in Walzer's own words, "that what was necessary and right was also wrong."[10] Such a conclusion brings ethics itself into a state of emergency or distress, and Walzer's otherwise highly regarded study has been criticized for it.[11]

Coherent and consistent moral reasoning on the British decision to bomb German cities would, if just-war norms are really binding, press one to the conclusion which John C. Ford reached while the war was still being fought:

> If anyone were to declare that modern war is necessarily total, and necessarily involves direct attack on the life of innocent civilians and, therefore, that obliteration bombing is justified, my reply would be: So much the worse for modern war. If it necessarily includes such means it is necessarily immoral itself.[12]

Although Walzer does not believe that all modern war is necessarily total, his book seems to suggest that when the defense of truly fundamental values can be achieved only through the violation of moral norms, we should say "so much the worse for morality." Supreme emergency seems to provide temporary license to go "beyond good and evil"; that is, it grants license to commit immoral acts in the defense of the truly basic values of civilizations. Supreme emergency confronts us with a fundamental moral antinomy or aporia in which we cannot seek justice without performing injustice, or in which we cannot remain just without allowing injustice to destroy the very foundations of a just society.

Walzer's position on the saturation bombing of World War II is consequently imbued with a deep sense of tragedy. He struggles mightily to hedge it around with stringent limits in an attempt to prevent the principle of noncombatant immunity from becoming another casualty of modern war. As Lawrence Freedman and others have pointed out, however, the doctrines that have governed plans for the use of nuclear weapons had their origins in the pre-Hiroshima theories on the strategic use of air power that led to bomber attacks on cities.[13] From a moral point of view, the key debates about the morality of the use of nuclear weapons through much of the nuclear age has a shape similar to that of the debate about the legitimacy of these bombardments of cities with conventional weapons. It is undoubtedly true that the advent of nuclear weapons in 1945 and their subsequent development must be regarded as a qualitative transition in the moral problem of warfare.[14] Nevertheless, the decision to resort to strategic bombardment during World War II provided a precedent for the development of strategies of counterpopulation nuclear warfare. In his critique of Walzer's argument from supreme emergency—a critique that is directed at Walzer because his position represents the most analytically precise version of a view held by a number of others—Stephen Lammers highlights the significance of this moral (or immoral) precedent:

It is true that politics includes single, unrepeated acts, the effects of which are quite limited. Politics also includes policy decisions which are implemented over time and which, when implemented, take on a life of their own. . . . In politics, a policy decision may lead to the creation of a social practice which becomes part of political life in the future. The evil that was supposed to be done at a given time may live on long after the conditions which made the policy "necessary" are past. Thus an evil determinate in kind may become indeterminate in duration.[15]

In fact, this is just what has happened to the temporary suspension of the principle of noncombatant immunity since World War II. Although there have been repeated efforts to provide alternatives to counterpopulation threats, the ultimate threat to attack cities has remained a permanent feature of the plans and the strategies of the nuclear powers. It is indeed fortunate that these strategies have not yet been carried into action; nevertheless, the mainstream version of nuclear strategy has continued to rely on a threat to violate this basic principle of the just-war tradition.

The dilemma posed by these strategies is evident in the discussions of nuclear deterrence in the recent European bishops' statements. Once again, however, Walzer's writing has the advantage of making this dilemma more explicit than do either the French or German bishops. He argues forcefully that the threat to attack civilians is itself immoral, even when this threat is part of a strategy of deterrence. It embodies a "commitment of murder."[16] Although he acknowledges that the threat to kill the innocent and the carrying out of this threat are very different things, they are very close on the level of intention. Counterpopulation deterrence—mutual assured destruction (MAD), for example—must therefore be judged morally perverted even if it succeeds in preventing the outbreak of war. Here, however, what Lammers is worried about becomes most relevant: once noncombatant immunity is set aside in a situation of supreme emergency, a social practice is legitimated that will be very difficult to delegitimate in the future. This is so because technological capacities and ideological rivalries have created social conditions in which the great nuclear adversaries of today feel supremely threatened, and this threat bodes to be of indeterminate duration. As Walzer puts it:

Supreme emergency has become a permanent condition. Deterrence is a way of coping with that condition, and though it is a bad way, there may be no other that is practical in a world of sovereign and suspicious states. We threaten evil in order not to do it, and the doing of it would be so terrible that the threat seems in comparison to be morally defensible.[17]

Here the same questions must be put to Walzer's approach to the ethics of deterrence that were raised concerning his legitimation of the early saturation bombing attacks of World War II. Is it based on a utilitarian moral theory, or is it really a suspension of morality itself? If the former is the case, he must bid adieu to the principle of noncombatant immunity as a relevant moral criterion in the current nuclear debate. Such an outcome would undermine his entire project of rethinking and developing the just-war tradition as an expression of a human rights ethic. If, on the other hand, he sees it as a suspension of morality, then there is little point in discussing the ethics of nuclear strategy at all. In either case, a wide chasm has been opened up between the traditional ethics of warfare and the contemporary policy arguments. Walzer sees no way out of this: "Nuclear weapons explode the theory of just war. They are the first of mankind's technological innovations that are simply not encompassable within the familiar moral world."[18] Unless an alternative can be found to this situation, ethics itself will succumb to the incubus of nuclear distress.

The Pacifist Alternative

There are two different kinds of possible response to this distressing analysis. Both call for recasting the presuppositions that lead Walzer and the European bishops to adopt this questionable emergency ethic. The first calls for an abandonment of the presupposition that moral responsibility necessarily demands the taking up of the burdens of political responsibility. This position is, broadly speaking, pacifist and sectarian. It is represented in the current debate by theologians such as John Howard Yoder and Stanley Hauerwas. The second alternative rests on the view that the situation of distress created by nuclear weapons can be transformed by replacing deterrence based on the threat to attack population centers with deterrence based on a credible, counterforce war-fighting capacity. This alternative appears today in a variety of versions, represented by moral and strategic thinkers such as James Johnson, Albert Wohlstetter, and William O'Brien.

The pacifism of Hauerwas and Yoder is based on an interpretation of the religious foundations of Christianity in the story of the people of Israel and the life, teaching, death, and resurrection of Jesus Christ. No moral thought that claims to be Christian can have any other ultimate basis. It is clear, however, that Hauerwas's version of an ethic of nonviolence is also based on an interpretation of our contemporary social, intellectual, and political situation. It is this latter interpretation that has led him to the conclusion that it is quite literally impossible to embody the ethical meaning of the Christian story in the political institutions and cultural patterns of modern Western society.

Here Hauerwas relies heavily on the reading of the development of modern Western intellectual and social history proposed by Alasdair MacIntyre, a philosopher who, though not religious himself, shares a strong sensitivity to the traditions of Western religious thought. In MacIntyre's view, post-Enlightenment ideas and institutions have destroyed the possibility of giving any universally plausible and rational account of the foundation of morality. He describes our situation today as one in which moral language is frequently used in public debate, but this usage is most often to express disagreement. There seems to be "no rational way of securing moral agreement in our culture."[19] As an example of moral disagreement for which there seems no terminus, MacIntyre cites the debate between those who regard the threat of nuclear war as a reason that we all ought to be pacifists today and those who argue that we must be prepared to fight nuclear war if we wish to maintain peace. The impossibility of adjudicating these disagreements is the result of the fact "that modern moral utterance and practice can only be understood as a series of fragmented survivals from an older past and that the insoluble problems which they have generated for modern moral theorists remain insoluble until this is well understood."[20] We have lost a coherent moral vision as a result of the culturally fragmenting effect of modernity, and we have also lost the kind of coherent institutions of communal life that are necessary to sustain such a vision.

MacIntyre regards the present situation as a kind of "new dark ages," and he prescribes a remedy that is analogous to the creation of monasticism and the revived emphasis on virtuous life in community during the dying years of the Roman Empire:

> What matters at this stage is the construction of local forms of community within which civility and the intellectual and moral life can be sustained through the new dark ages which are already upon us. And

if the tradition of the virtues was able to survive the horrors of the last dark ages, we are not entirely without grounds for hope. This time however the barbarians are not waiting beyond the frontiers; they have been governing us for quite some time. And it is our lack of consciousness of this that constitutes part of our predicament. We are not waiting for Godot, but for another—doubtless very different—St. Benedict.[21]

Although the cogency of MacIntyre's interpretation of our intellectual and social history need not detain us here (in my view it has both strengths and weaknesses), it is clear why Hauerwas appeals to it as a secular, philosophical warrant for the revival of a form of Christian sectarian pacifism. The "explosion" of the just-war theory is the result of the head-on collision of the principle of noncombatant immunity, which is rooted in a theory of human rights, with the principle of proportionality, which calls for the comparative weighing of relative goods and evils. The collision is evident in Walzer's writings, where a human rights–based just-war theory conflicts with a form of utilitarianism in the situation of supreme emergency. It has become impossible to reconcile these two principles as long as our world is one where threats against populations are deterred by proportionate counterthreats of the same sort. Discrimination and proportionality in the present circumstances are but "fragmented survivals" uprooted from the moral tradition in which they initially germinated by the force of modern political and military realities.

The tradition that gave rise to classical just-war theory shares a common presupposition with the pacifist perspective Hauerwas advocated. The common ground on which just-war theory and pacifism stand is the conviction that survival—even the survival of the most fundamental of this-worldly values—is not an absolute value.[22] Both the biblical eschatology that sees the kingdom of God as the ultimate reference point for ethical choice and the Christianized version of the Aristotelian teleological ethic developed by Thomas Aquinas relativize intrawordly values. They envision the possibility that these values may sometimes have to be sacrificed. Fidelity to the call of the kingdom of God or to the teleological ordering of human nature to union with God can come into conflict with the political values of justice and human rights in ultimately tragic circumstances, and these later values must sometimes give way.

It is fair to say, I think, that neither social contract theory nor utilitarianism shares this perspective. For example, a perpetual problem with social contract theories has been the difficulty of providing reasons that the contract should be kept when doing so will subvert the reasons that support the obligations to adhere to the contract in the first place—that is, universal protection of freedom and enlightened self-interest, including my own.[23] At the same time, contract theory cannot advance cogent reasons why the contract should be broken, for to do so would also deny the universally normative rationality on which it rests. This bind is evident in Walzer's conclusion that the suspension of noncombatant immunity in the supreme emergency is both right and wrong at the same time.

This sort of problem inevitably arises when an ethic is based on universal, rational principles that lack an eschatological or teleological point of reference. Both contract theory and utilitarianism force us into antinomies where we simply cannot know what we ought to do, not because of lack of social or political knowledge, but because of the limits of the moral theories themselves. The upshot is an increased fragmentation of the human moral community as diverse solutions are asserted from different quarters. Hauerwas concludes, therefore, that modern intellectual categories and social institutions make it impossible to develop an argument about the morality of nuclear strategy that has a chance of universal acceptance. He believes we must be prepared to accept the "dividedness" of the world, even on this fundamental moral level. He goes farther than MacIntyre here, for it is not simply the loss of an Aristotelian teleological framework that has brought this dividedness about. From a Christian perspective, it must be this way, since the hope for a reconciled world is necessarily eschatological—it can be realized only beyond history. Therefore, the quest for a universal set of moral norms that can order a divided community in accord with reason is illusory.[24]

One can therefore interpret Hauerwas as implying that *all* contemporary normative ethical systems are in some sense sectarian. Or, better, there is no universal moral rationality to opt out of as the Troeltschian typology suggests "sect-type" religious groups are wont to do. All moral traditions are history bound and tied to the narratives and traditions of the communities that form them. Therefore, Christian pacifism cannot be charged with being morally deficient because it does not propose a political ethic capable of regulating the life of society as a whole on the basis of universal rational principles. In Hauerwas's view, all the competing normative visions available are subject to this charge as well. In addition, Christian pacifism has a distinct advantage over those systems that would justify violence for the enforcement of a partial ethical vision. It does not claim to be operating on the basis of universal rationality, but it acknowledges that it is shaped by a particular narrative tradition: the story of Israel and of Jesus Christ. It does not abandon the *hope* for universal reconciliation and the full achievement of justice and peace in society, but it regards this hope as eschatological and to be fulfilled by the action of God, not by human force of arms.

Neither does this sort of Christian pacifism believe that all normative visions are equally true. Rather, it holds that the ethics of nonviolence is in fact the true perspective, and that this truth is verified in the experience of the nonviolent community. Such a concrete historical experience of justice and peace in community is in fact the only basis for judging the truth or falsity of normative frameworks. Thus convincing those with other convictions to change their stance can be done only by inviting them to share this experience and providing an alternative community in which this experience is available to them. As Hauerwas puts it:

> We have no guarantee, of course, that others will accept such a way of life, but Christians must live with the confidence that others will find that such a life frees them from the fears that give birth to slavery and injustice. God has promised the church that if we are faithful our life will not be without effect. The church's task does not depend on nor is it sustained by such effectiveness, however; it is sustained by our experience that by living faithfully we do find God in the truth of our existence.[25]

This, I take it, is the sort of thing MacIntyre has in mind when he says that modern society, living under the threat of insoluble moral conflicts, is waiting for a new St. Benedict.

I have discussed Hauerwas and MacIntyre at some length for two reasons. Their interrelated viewpoints are a relatively sophisticated reflection of an attitude that is increasingly present on the popular level of the nuclear debate—namely, that it is next to impossible consistently to relate moral norms to today's highly complex strategic arguments. For Hauerwas and MacIntyre, that is simply a particular case of the problem of relating moral norms to a form of rationality that has lost its teleological connection with ends and its religious connection with eschatological hope. On this level I am in full agreement with them. This is not to say that morality is impossible without religion (an issue that I prefer to leave to another occasion). Rather, it reflects a conviction that a loss of a sense of the historical possibilities for changing the present terms of the debate leads to an ethical dead end. Teleological and eschatological dimensions in ethics keep this from happening as neither social contract theory nor utilitarianism can do. An ethic that starts and ends within the boundaries of the present conflict-ridden situation cannot fail to lead to insoluble puzzles. Ethics is meant to transform the human condition from what it is to what it could be, not simply to help us better understand the conflicting values of our world. For this reason I welcome the challenge from this quarter.

The second reason for considering this approach is to criticize it constructively in the hope of moving the debate on the relation of morality and nuclear policy to a more fruitful level. Despite Hauerwas's strong desire to move us out of the present bind by his appeal to an eschatological hope, he lacks principles that can guide policy in a historically incremental way. His view goes beyond an "ethics of distress" to the proclamation of the death of political ethics as this term is normally understood. This is because Hauerwas, in contrast to Augustine and Paul Ramsey, rejects the value of norms for distinguishing between more and less perfect forms of justice and peace in the earthly city.[26] He draws a stark contrast between the absolute peace and justice of the kingdom of God and the injustice and violence of the world of power politics. For Ramsey, following Augustine, the picture is considerably more complex than this.

In Augustine and Ramsey, the city of God and the earthly city cannot be identified with distinct communities in history—for example, the church and the Roman Empire or a contemporary pacifist community and the superpowers. The two "cities" coexist in all things human, whether these be nation-states, churches, or even individuals. The ethical task, then, is transformation, not a division into sheep and goats. And it is the norms of the just-war tradition that guide us as we seek this transformation of a world that is a mixture of good and evil. This tradition situates conflict in a historical, developmental framework and demands that we seize every opportunity to further this transformation, while recognizing that it will always be incomplete within history. This Augustinian perspective, in other words, does not deny the moral tensions inherent in political life, but it does refuse to allow tension to become dualism or to explode into self-contradiction.

Ethics and Limited War

This transformationist Augustinian interpretation of political ethics and just-war theory may provide a clue to how we can move beyond the distressing state of the current debate on the relation of morality and nuclear war. The explosion of the just war-theory described by Walzer is the result of the presence of immoral intentions in MAD deterrence theories. The strategic debates of the 1960s had sought to find an alternative to this sort of deterrence by proposing a variety of counterforce strategies that could in fact serve as a credible deterrent without threatening to attack civilians directly. That debate, Walzer concludes, petered out in the mid-1960s when the extent of collateral damage to civilians by most imaginable counterforce attacks and the high likelihood of escalation of any superpower conflict to a catastrophic nuclear war became clear.[27] Walzer's conclusion in 1977 was similar to the one reached more recently by Lawrence Freedman:

> The position we have reached is one where stability depends on something that is more the antithesis of strategy than its apotheosis—on threats that things will get out of hand, that we might act irrationally, that possibly through inadvertence we could set in motion a process that in its development and conclusion would be beyond human control and comprehension.[28]

Nuclear strategy is a mixture of good intentions and evil threats. It is a construct of human rationality that "works" only because of our fear that human beings will act irrationally and immorally. Its consequences might be peace of a sort, a catastrophic war, or a long twilight struggle of uncertainty and doubt.

Nuclear strategy, we might say, is a quintessentially Augustinian phenomenon. It is virtually impossible to untangle the good and the evil elements in it. The good is an aspect of the evil, and the evil both the source and the possible outcome of the good it seeks to achieve. Just as Augustine's well-known robber bands had their own form of justice, so the darkness of nuclear strategy does contain a measure of rational purpose within it. But they *were* robbers, and the strategy remains full of demonic potential. We cannot simply accept it, nor can we simply reject it. The pacifist risks the loss of the good it can achieve by making aversion to the evil in it the sole basis of decision. Walzer and the European bishops are more cautious because their basic adherence to just-war tradition has given them a more Augustinian political sensibility. They recognize that rejection of deterrence could have a terrible price, and their acceptance of it is reluctant and even tortured. They call for the creation of alternatives to a system that seeks to "win the peace" by threatening civilian populations. But neither really says much about what these alternatives might be. This is understandable in Walzer's case, I believe, because the alternatives that are currently being proposed were still in gestation as he wrote his book. I am less willing to grant the French bishops this excuse, for when they wrote their letter in 1983 a wide array of alternatives to MAD not only were under discussion but were being translated into policy. As Stanley Hoffmann has noted, the French bishops seem insufficiently aware of the new technologies and strategic doctrines that make counterforce deterrence and defense the moral point at issue in the current debate.[29] By provisionally legitimating countervalue deterrence, they not only acquiesce in the explosion of the just-war theory, but also, because they do not take the newer strategic proposals into account, implicitly legitimate policies they seem not to have considered. The lack of attention to the specifics of these new strategic doctrines is also a problem with the German bishops' document, although I suspect the reasons for it were more political than in the case of the French.

The Augustinian view of political ethics should put us on guard against this sort of reluctance to take seriously the concrete possibilities of changing the dangerous situation we are in. Augustinian thinking does not expect to be able to untangle all the moral threads of political life. But it is equally insistent that history is an open system, capable of change and movement. The way we respond to the openings for the enhancement of justice and community among peoples and for the reduction of injustice and violence is an index of whether our polity is simply a band of murderers and robbers or something better than this. MAD seeks to establish a form of justice, but it is the justice of a murderous world. The issue is this: What can be done to transform it?

It is here that the various counterforce nuclear strategies under consideration today demand scrutiny from a moral perspective. I have argued elsewhere that it is impossible to reach moral conclusions about nuclear deterrence and defense in the abstract.[30] It is the abstraction from actual and concrete policy choices that induces the internal emergency or distress within ethics itself. If we fail to consider actual concrete alternatives to the morally self-contradictory strategy of MAD, we foreclose the possibility that ethical principles can transform the situation into one that is less dangerous and more just.

It is precisely this search for alternatives that can be found in contemporary discussions of whether there is a possibility of creating a strategy for the deterrence of war through a credible, counterforce threat that would itself meet the norms of discrimination and proportionality proposed by the just-war theory. The advocates of such limited nuclear war strategies all admit that there is a grave level of uncertainty over whether these limits would in fact be respected should deterrence fail. They differ in how they actually conceive these limits. Albert Wohlstetter believes that targets should be limited to the military and that strict limits on collateral civilian damage are necessary. Colin Gray would expand these limits to include the military and political leadership of the adversary, an expansion that renders a "decapitating" first strike at least imaginable. William V. O'Brien stretches the limits even further, when he argues that strategic attacks on cities could conceivably be part of a "limited" war where they were carried out for purposes of intrawar deterrence—that is, as a means of dissuading an adversary from taking further escalating steps that will likely lead to holocaust.[31]

In considering these proposals for moving away from MAD and toward a strategy that seeks to adhere to just-war norms, the problem is evident: the boundaries between counterforce and countervalue strategies are very tenuous indeed. We seem almost inevitably pushed to the conclusion, reached by Walzer and Freedman, that any sort of deterrence works only because of the fear that things will get out of control. In my view, the proposals of both Colin Gray and William O'Brien are virtually indistinguishable from MAD. If actually carried out, both seem certain to produce a form of spasmodic or indiscriminate response and counter-response that would be impossible to distinguish from the failure of MAD. The danger of both proposals is increased by the fact that both Gray's decapitation strategies and O'Brien's limited-war proposals depend on the deployment of first-strike-capable weapons—a sure formula for making deterrence less stable. Therefore, neither of them, in my view, really represents the desired transformation of our political/military circumstances in accord with the Augustinian imperative. Both leave the situation of distress much as it was.

The case of Wohlstetter is more complex. His statement that we must "face up to evasions making 'murder respectable' in such chaste phrases as 'countervalue attacks' " seems clearly to rule out O'Brien's rather expansive version of the nature of limited war.[32] His view that Soviet leaders value military power as much as they do civilian populations has analogies with Colin Gray's emphasis on the value of political control in the Soviet system, a valuation that leads Gray to think that threat of decapitation will be such a strong deterrent to Soviet adventures. Wohlstetter does not seem to advocate this approach, but neither does he rule it out. His real concern is that MAD not only is an immoral strategy but is actually incredible as a deterrent, because it rests on an insane threat to commit suicide. His desire to develop a limited-war strategy as an alternative to MAD is supported by both moral and political reason. In this he is on solid Augustinian ground.

One of the chief problems with his approach, however, is his tendency to identify "minimum deterrence" with MAD. This use of language, which is not Wohlstetter's creation, introduces a conceptual confusion into the contemporary debate. It suggests that *increases in our war-fighting capacity* necessarily move us away from the specter of mutual destruction. This is not necessarily so. In fact, it may have the opposite effect, depending on *what kind* of war-fighting capacities are developed. For example, the Scowcroft commission proposed the development and deployment of both the MX and single-warhead mobile missiles. These two systems are both war-fighting weapons, designed for deterrence through a credible threat. But the threat posed by the two weapons to an adversary is significantly different. In my view, the replacement of MIRVed Minuteman missiles with the single-warhead mobile missile would be a step toward a "more minimal" deterrent than the one we now have, whereas MX is a move toward a "more maximal" one, if *minimal* and *maximal* are used to refer to the dangers they present. This would still entail a severe danger that nuclear war could occur. But the danger would be less than under the present arrangement and much less than in the world of vulnerable first-strike weapons we are moving into. Wohlstetter's polemic against minimal deterrence needs to be refined by distinctions like these. One can also ask: do not such distinctions enable us to imagine ways that large numbers of currently deployed nuclear weapons in our supposedly minimal deterrent could be replaced by conventional forces, including conventionally armed precision-guided missiles. Wohlstetter himself suggests this, but I would be much happier if he had more carefully explored the possible meanings of minimal deterrence before accepting the convention of identifying the idea with MAD. Such an exploration could open the way for us to seize opportunities to transform the grossly murderous logic of present strategy into something that is at least less murderous if not truly pacific.

In my opinion, this is the avenue that the U.S. Catholic bishops have taken in the pastoral letter *The Challenge of Peace*. This is not the place for a detailed analysis of this complex document.[33] One point, however, is notable in the context of this discussion. The U.S. bishops do not advocate minimal deterrence in the sense Wohlstetter presupposed—that is, MAD. Indeed, they oppose it vigorously: "it is not morally acceptable to intend to kill the innocent as part of a strategy of deterring nuclear war."[34] At the same time they argue against forms of deterrence that will increase the danger of nuclear war or that target military forces in ways that are likely to produce disproportionate collateral damage:

> While we welcome any effort to protect civilian populations, we do not want to legitimize or encourage moves which extend deterrence beyond the specific objectives of preventing the use of nuclear weapons or other actions which could lead directly to a nuclear exchange.[35]

With these criteria as background, they consider specific alternatives to MAD and their implications for the quest for the goals of nuclear war prevention and the defense of justice and human rights.

The U.S. bishops' specific conclusions are an attempt to direct policy into avenues that are less dangerous than some of the war-fighting strategies being proposed (for example, that of Colin Gray); less open ended than others (for example, those of Wohlstetter); and less inconsistent with just-war norms than a third type of limited-war doctrine (for example, those of O'Brien). The conclusions they draw are largely negative: no "hard-target kill weapons, no protracted war scenarios, no quest for superiority, no systems which make disarmament more difficult to achieve." They also make a number of positive recommendations, largely in the areas of the need for negotiated arms control treaties; removal of nuclear forces from forward-based positions in Europe; and improved command, control, and communication systems.[36]

Some have argued that the U.S. bishops have moved to a level of specificity that goes beyond their competence as moral teachers in making recommendations of this sort. On the contrary, attending to the actual proposals being made today is really the *only* way to reach conclusions about the relation of morality to nuclear strategy. To argue against this level of specificity in addressing nuclear questions would be analogous to saying that moral teachers should speak about the morality of medicine but should never discuss any specific medical procedure. This would be absurd, for there is no such thing as the morality of medicine as such. One could say, of course, that if there had never been a fall from grace by Adam and Eve, there would be no sickness and death in our world, as Genesis, St. Paul, and the Christian tradition have long taught. But in a fallen and divided world, sickness exists, doctors are needed, and ethical perspectives on their practice are a legitimate concern of theologians, philosophers, and bishops, not just of the physicians themselves. The same can be said of the ethics of warfare. It depends on an analysis of the pathways that are open to us for healing political conflict and avoiding actions that make the illness worse.

In my view, the U.S. bishops have done as good a job as anyone has in synthesizing the religious, philosophical, political, and military dimensions of the nuclear issue. There are, however, limits to their achievement. In particular, I think more needs to be said about defensive systems and the various types of weapons proposed as replacements for MIRVed missiles. Can any of these serve the purposes of minimal deterrence as the term has been redefined here—that is, as minimally dangerous? Despite these limits, the U.S. bishops' letter serves as an example of moral reasoning that seeks to avoid the self-contradiction of the "ethics of distress." As good practitioners of Augustinian moral theory, they seek to transform and redeem a broken polis by seizing those opportunities for peace, order, and justice that history has given us today. Although their work hardly closes the debate, it does provide a model for avoiding some of the dead ends into which we have wandered.

Notes

1. "The French Bishops' Statement: Winning Peace," *Origins* 13, no. 26 (December 8, 1983): 442, 443, 443 n. 20.

2. Joint Pastoral Letter of the German Bishops, *Out of Justice, Peace* (Dublin: Irish Messenger Publications, 1983), 61, 39.

3. Ibid., 61.

4. Ibid.

5. Ibid., 61–62.

6. Thomas Aquinas, *Summa Theologiae*, Ia IIae q.91, art. 2.

7. Michael Walzer, *Just and Unjust Wars: A Moral Argument with Historical Illustrations* (New York: Basic Books, 1977), 129, 153, 133.

8. Ibid., 252.

9. Ibid., 260, 323.

10. Ibid., 324.

11. See, for example, the recent study by Stephen E. Lammers, "Area Bombing in World War II: The Argument of Michael Walzer," *Journal of Religious Ethics* 111 (1983): 96–113.

12. John C. Ford, S.J., "The Morality of Obliteration Bombing," *Theological Studies* 5 (1944): 268.

13. Lawrence Freedman, *The Evolution of Nuclear Strategy* (New York: St. Martin's Press, 1981), 3ff.

14. For a helpful discussion of some of the dimensions of this qualitative transition, see Michael Howard, "Bombing and the Bomb," in his *Studies in War and Peace* (New York: Viking Press, 1971), 141–53.

15. Lammers, "Area Bombing," 104.

16. Walzer, *Just and Unjust Wars*, 272.

17. Ibid., 274.

18. Ibid., 282.

19. Alasdair MacIntyre, *After Virtue: A Study in Moral Theory* (Notre Dame, Ind.: University of Notre Dame Press, 1981), 6.

20. Ibid., 104–5.

21. Ibid., 244–45.

22. See Stanley Hauerwas, "On Surviving Justly: An Ethical Analysis of Nuclear Disarmament," in Jill Raitt, ed., *Religious Conscience and Nuclear Warfare* (1982 Paine Lectures in Religion, privately printed by the University of Missouri–Columbia), 19.

23. For a helpful discussion of this, see Ronald Green, *Religious Reason: The Rational and Moral Basis of Religious Belief* (New York: Oxford University Press, 1978), ch. 3.

24. See Stanley Hauerwas, *A Community of Character* (Notre Dame, Ind.: University of Notre Dame Press, 1981), 101.

25. Ibid., 106.

26. See Paul Ramsey, *War and the Christian Conscience: How Shall Modern War Be Conducted Justly?* (Durham, N.C.: Duke University Press, 1961), chs. 2, 3.

27. Walzer, *Just and Unjust Wars*, 278.

28. Freedman, *Nuclear Strategy*, 400.

29. Stanley Hoffmann, "Le cri d'alarme de l'église américaine," *Le monde* (November 19, 1983), 1.

30. David Hollenbach, S.J., *Nuclear Ethics: A Christian Moral Argument* (New York: Paulist Press, 1983), 73–77.

31. See Wohlstetter's reply to his critics in "Morality and Deterrence: Wohlstetter and Critics," *Commentary* (December 1983), 13–22; Colin Gray and Keith Payne, "Victory Is Possible," *Foreign Policy* 39 (Summer 1980): 14–27; and William V. O'Brien, *The Conduct of Just and Limited War* (New York: Praeger, 1981), 135.

32. Albert Wohlstetter, "Optimal Ways to Confuse Ourselves," *Foreign Policy* 20 (Autumn 1975): 198.

33. For several views of it, see Philip J. Murnion, ed., *Catholics and Nuclear War: A*

Commentary on "The Challenge of Peace," The U.S. Catholic Bishops' Pastoral Letter on War and Peace (New York: Crossroad, 1983); and Michael Novak, *Moral Clarity in the Nuclear Age* (Nashville, Tenn.: Thomas Nelson, 1983).

34. National Conference of Catholic Bishops, *The Challenge of Peace: God's Promise and Our Response* (Washington, D.C.: United States Catholic Conference, 1983), par. 178.

35. Ibid., par. 185.

36. Ibid., pars. 188–90, 191.

4 • Bluff or Revenge: The Watershed in Democratic Deterrence Awareness

JOHN HOWARD YODER

For centuries it was the claim of Catholic just-war tradition that it provided a usable set of tools to make applicable distinctions among available political options. It claimed to do so by integrating a multiplicity of themes and modes of moral reasoning. It incorporated consequential modes of moral reasoning, taking account of real possibilities, weighing the foreseeable effects of responsible action. It incorporated ontologically founded deontological modes of reasoning based on the nature of man, the nature of the nation, the sacredness of life, and the conviction that certain deeds may be intrinsically identifiable as in the category of *malum in se*. To those it added empirically derived readings about the decision-making situation—last resort, legality, and winnability.

All of this proceeded with relative confidence in the pastoral and political wisdom of episcopacy as a social structure and in the adequacy of "Christian natural law insight"[1] as a mental method, to keep all of these factors operative in the mix, and never to sin seriously against any of them. A proper understanding of this properly dosed mixing could be trusted, it was thought, to defend us (1) against a purely quantifying consequentialism that authorizes people to do any evil with a good conscience as long as they can claim that someone else was going to do worse; and (2) against a pragmatic consequentialism with a bad conscience, justifying as "necessary sin" deeds one knows to be intrinsically evil.

If we are to honor the moral integrity in the original intent of the just-war tradition from Ambrose to Vitoria and Grotius, we must resist the temptation to boil down the multidimensional mix to less worthy simplifications that respect fewer of the variables.

The new shape of the theme of deterrence is a good test of how the just-war tradition is intended to work. This is not the case for all past usage of the threat of violent sanctions to prevent evil deeds. Such threats have always existed, and it has always been thinkable that they be handled within the regular casuistry of the just-war tradition, even though a particular concept was not actually *named* "deterring."

What is new in the present conjuncture is the use for deterrent effect of a threat whose actual execution would overreach necessarily the barriers of discrimination, proportionality, and/or noncombatant immunity. The pure form of this new problem is obviously the massive or all-out use of nuclear weapons. The fruitfulness of this question, its urgency, and its need for clarification are not diminished by our not being clear at just what point massive begins.

The intent of this analysis is both to make some progress in the interpretation of what must actually be done about deterrence by means of the progressive clarification of the just-war theory and to learn about the limits of the just-war tradition by asking how its resources are strained by the concrete case of deterrence.

What is the inner moral logic of a threat that one hopes not to have to carry out? If such hope is rooted in a firm moral rejection of the carrying out as always necessarily wrong, and if we all know this to be the case, it is hard to avoid a posture of "bluff," i.e., a threat which one knows one cannot carry out but hopes the enemy will nonetheless fear. If the carrying out is on the other hand not firmly excluded, then the readiness to carry out the threat after it has failed to deter becomes morally odd. The following points must be considered:

1. Carrying out the threat after it has failed to deter can no longer be justified as deterring. Now it must be thought of as retaliation. Yet this can no longer be justified by any of the reasons whereby just-war thinking in the past has made a case for reprisal.
2. It can be revenge; yet revenge is not morally justified in any framework except that of a theocratic holy war, and then on the grounds of special revelation. It has no place in modern Western just-war thinking, and no consequentially justifiable social effect.
3. Going through with the counterattack can be intended to prove that the bluff was no bluff, but that proof no longer has the function which was supposed to justify it in the first place. The additional destruction is henceforth gratuitous.
4. It cannot be justified on any consequential grounds that begin by taking stock of the shape of the universe after having undergone the

massive first attack which the threat failed to deter. The counterattack will not bring the victim of the massive first strike closer to anything that could be called "winning." It will bring the world, including one's own civilization, closer to destruction either through permanent nuclear winter or through radiation diseases, even where the bombs themselves did not destroy.

It is thus no surprise that, with the passage of time, social and intellectual pressures have moved people either toward admitting the moral possibility of a first strike, thereby abandoning the claim that deterrence is justified by its success in that the weapons would never have to be used, or on the other side toward a rising readiness to run risks by granting the moral imperative of nuclear pacifism, even before there is at hand an alternative political recourse that could promise to save all of the values national preparedness claims to be saving.

The closer one looks at this picture, the more difficult it becomes to sustain a moral argument that will not slip off the razor's edge into either readiness to wage nuclear war after all on one hand, or the obligation to renounce the weapon on the other. Staying on the razor's edge increasingly approximates what some have called the "bluff." By this is meant the hope that the threat of nuclear retaliation will continue to be effective as a restraining influence on Soviet policy without our having to claim that we are ready to justify morally the use of the weapons. To threaten overtly something that one does not plan to do is sometimes called bluffing. Bluffing in cards, however, usually means pretending to have a weapon one does not have. In this case, however, it is very clear that we do have the weapon. Then the notion that one might pretend to be preparing to fire it, while one really does not have that intention, is a much more complex pose. It can be doubted that such a stance is possible at all in a democratic society, although it might be more thinkable in a dictatorial one. This possibility is also quite dubious within a bureaucratic military organization, where many decisions are delegated to field officers operating within previously established scenario provisions. Perhaps this would be easier to conceive of in a system where the tactical decisions are made at the top. In both these respects, the Soviet system might be more capable of a credible bluff than is ours.

Having stated the question and seen why it is worthy of analysis, we move to the most prominent recent instance of its being handled in public, namely in 1983 Roman Catholic bishops' pastoral letter *The Challenge of Peace*. The bishops make quite clear, on the grounds that have come to be designated as "nuclear pacifism," that no massive use of nuclear weapons can ever be morally justified. They simplify the question and harden their thesis by their empirical reading, according to which escalation is practically inevitable, so that any initiation of nuclear combat beyond the "firebreak" is tantamount to having decided in favor of an all-out strike. Whether this reading of the inevitability of escalation is empirically correct, the present analysis need not evaluate.

What then remains of the morality of threatening that prohibited use?

The bishops avoid speaking directly to guide policy makers who currently would have to answer that question as part of their public responsibility. They do not say to the president or to the joint chiefs of staff that they should state that they will not commit the intrinsically immoral act of firing our nuclear arsenal. They thereby avoid any open form of what some have called "bluff," the threat whose implementation one subjectively knows is excluded.

One of the participants in the bishops' drafting process said in my hearing, "If deterrence should fail, then we would have to decide what to do next. We will cross that bridge when we come to it." It is quite doubtful that "crossing that bridge when we come to it" is a possible scenario of how command decisions would be made after a nuclear attack, or of how the bishops could be consulted under such circumstances. The whole point of ethical deliberation and public political deliberation about matters of ethical import is that (1) they need to be thought about ahead of time because there is too little time to think during the situation; and (2) they need to be thought of ahead of time because they will be decided not by individuals on the spur of the moment but by institutional processes that are already rolling. If we do not thoroughly explore before the attack all available alternative responses, it would seem that only a naive occasionalism would hold open any hope that decisions made after the attack would take account of the moral insight we have already expressed.

The bishops thus had to take a different path. They transformed the question from one of concrete decision into one of timing. They said that intrinsically the possession of those arms is unacceptable, but that it may be conditionally and transitionally condoned on the way to their abolition by means of negotiating processes for which their temporary possession may be essential. In the second draft of the letter the bishops had said this in terms of tolerating an evil for a good end, but they were reminded by theologians that such a phrase would be counter to one of the simplest classical rules of morality in Catholic tradition, namely that one must not do an evil deed, even a lesser one, directly and intentionally for the sake of good.

So the third draft of the letter made what looks to the layperson like the same point but in other wording. They thereby produced a rough analogy to what in European Protestant thinking since the late 1950s had been called "a time of grace." This meant that although we had been doing the wrong thing, God had preserved us, without our merit, from its danger, but that the time of God's patience is coming to an end and we must cease doing the wrong that God has thus far preserved us from having to pay for. Calling it grace meant that the claim could not be made that the MAD threats were justified by having worked. That we have made it this far means that God, not the system, is good. Both the current Catholic language of temporary concessions and the German Protestant language of grace are calculated to bring effective pressure for change upon those in power. They do not ask for the moon or for past commitments to be undone, but they do ask for fundamental change and believe that their calling for it should be credible because it is patient and not founded in a moral absolutism.

This kind of concession, by naming a condition that may not be taken for granted, has the merit of not claiming justification in principle. The second draft of the letter had made the conditional quality of this acquiescence clear by placing it in a time frame correlated with real political goals, namely by setting conditions that were possible to verify or falsify so as to discern that they had been met or had not been met. It did so by quoting an earlier statement. In congressional committee testimony in 1979 John Cardinal Krol had said that not only the use of strategic nuclear weapons but also the declared intent to use them is morally wrong:

> It is of the utmost importance that negotiations proceed to meaningful and continuing reductions . . . and eventually to the phasing out altogether of nuclear deterrence. . . . As long as there is hope of this occurring, Catholic moral teaching is willing, while negotiations proceed, to tolerate the possession of nuclear weapons for deterrence as the lesser of the two evils. If that hope were to disappear the moral attitude of the Catholic church would certainly have to shift to one of uncompromising condemnation of both use and possession of such weapons.[2]

This phrasing differs dramatically from most other evaluations. The readiness to condone present deterrent capacity is stated subject to verifiable or falsifiable conditions, the fulfilling of which can be measured in the real events of U.S. politics. Negotiations must be proceeding, and there must be hope of their succeeding, for this conditional acquiescence to be obtained. A warning is expressed: if these requirements are not met, acquiescence will have to be withdrawn and condemnation become stronger.

In this arrangement we may discern a classical instance of the pastoral/ political wisdom of episcopacy at its best. Without affirming the fundamental adequacy of consequentialist reasoning forms, the bishops accept such argument for the short run. They let stand a weapons system whose responsibly structured political purpose is the infliction of morally inadmissible damage on great numbers of enemy civilians. They let it stand because its stated purpose is to prevent the worst from happening. They thereby accept for the short range the scenario of the NATO authorities. Yet they seek to break the back of that consequentialism by placing it under a time bind. They challenge it to produce on its promise—to demonstrate its ability to deliver the projected consequences. If it can, we are all saved from the worst. If it cannot, then the conditional approbation which had been conceded to the entire deterrent enterprise is withdrawn. Thus an ethic of principle is still ultimately safe behind the surface acceptance of a policy based on calculated consequences. This is why the third and final drafts, dropping the Krol argument, must be seen as having stepped back from bindingness.

Perhaps the bishops were as honest as they could be in that they did not claim to resolve the tension, but rather left it dangling. But since it is dangling, so too is the credibility of the moral framework they say they are interpreting.

The bishops' letter does not claim that the compromise between the logic which would call for nuclear pacifism and the current toleration of deterrent capacity has been thought through and justified on the basis of general ethical principles. That is why I say that their reason is rather pastoral and political than systematic, i.e., it is more a matter of timing and patience in the midst of an incomplete conversation than it is a satisfying line of argument. I say this not by way of condemnation but rather as interpretation. It is an appropriate trait of pastoral wisdom not to press an uncomfortable new truth upon the faithful with simple "authority." It is quite honest to say, "If everyone had time to think things through, the only honest position would be nuclear pacifism, but the question is too new. We do not believe that we should jeopardize our ability to continue as shepherds of our faithful by seeking to impose this insight upon them without there being time for them to appropriate this insight validly." The paradox of pastoral patience is quite different from the confident and self-righteous paradox of an intellectual affirming at once of two contradictory lines of argument. Contrasted to an earlier age when bishops would make normative statements without consulting the faithful, this stance, which sketches the main lines of normative teaching and yet grants the teachers' inability to demand conformity to their teaching on the part of the unconvinced faithful—understandably unconvinced since the teaching is new—is worthy of respect. It is most worthy of respect when it grants most openly that it is not ethically consistent.

But pastoral wisdom is methodological open-endedness. Where the bishops avoided definition we must look elsewhere for illumination. We turn from contemporary pastoring to conceptual analysis. The first resort of Roman Catholic thought during the early generations of awareness of this problem has been to stretch the category of *intention* in order to sort out these matters. That cannot be held to have led to any firm clarification as yet. The new question is one with which the old language, even if one held that it had been adequate before, was not intended to help. When Thomas Aquinas used the term *intention* in his own just-war formulation, it was to designate the ultimate direction in which one hopes one's actions will move reality: the peace which is to be served by justified war is a better future state of the cosmos. Intention is objective, an historical goal. Thomas, however, quoted a passage from Augustine in which intention is a subjective attitude: a wrong "intention" is pride or hatred.

Neither of the above definitions will cover what is done with the word *intention* in its use in the doctrine of double effect. When one does evil to achieve good, according to double-effect theory, one distinguishes by an act of will between those consequences which one very well knows one will bring about but which one says one does not "intend," and other consequences, sufficiently desirable to outweigh the evil ones, which one does "intend." This mix of nuances of "intending" is an intrinsically odd kind of thought and action.

Leaning in the other direction, the standard line of thought inaugurated by Gertrude Anscombe seeks in a more integrated way to speak of "intention" as a whole, without reducing it to the action itself or the consequences of the action.[3]

No attempt shall be made here to sort out the proximate values of such definitional moves as they seek to help clarify issues and discern meaningful distinctions. There may be some value in locating one level of moral integrity in such a way that it cannot be disproved by any disparity between the will and the deed, whether due to moral weakness, to misinformation, to lack of effective control of the situation, or even to a temporary lapse into sloth, pride, or malevolence. If in any of these ways it is conceptually helpful to separate the intention from the act, we need not challenge such a use of intention. Yet none of these suffices to make the new distinctions clear and responsible which we are told must be made between institutionalizing the threat of nuclear annihilation and denying that one "intends" its execution. Nor does the pastoral letter claim that greater methodological clarity is the solution. That claim is rather made by their critics.

Michael Novak objected, against the entire line of analysis in the bishops' letter, that there is a more nuanced and refined intentionality thinking which *The Challenge of Peace* does not respect. He himself named three different levels or dimensions: fundamental, secondary, and objective, without showing us just how they related to one another. More important:

1. He gave no indication that this particular segregation of levels has any roots in Catholic moral thought.
2. He did not indicate what the effect of adopting it would be, whether to make more careful or less careful the shared exercise of moral discernment.
3. He did not clarify whether on any of the three levels the direct, intended, indiscriminate, and/or disproportionate killing of the innocent is justified. It would appear that if his argument were to deliver the conclusions he seemed to want—in favor of present administration policies—he would have had to approve of such murder on the second (secondary) and third (objective) of his three levels, while rejecting it on the first (fundamental).

The separation of levels has thus added nothing to the clarification of moral choices: it has merely located consequentialism in one compartment ("the choice of an immoral act which however prevents greater evil") and murder in another.[4]

In sum, the commonsense meaning of intention suggests that an action is more than an action, that a deed is the outworking of a disposition or purpose on the part of the agent. Some complexities of moral analysis, concerning the distance from willing to doing, may be illuminated by the notion. But does it help explain credible threatening to do what one may morally not do? Unfortunately, past elaboration of the notion of intention has been multidimensional and inclusive. For some the intention is more than the act: it imparts to a decision or an action a broader meaning, rooted in the character of the agent, or in the purposes to which the agent is committed, or in the community to which the agent belongs. The effect of that line of interpreation would be to decrease the leeway left in specific casuistic tight spots for choosing "lesser evil" adjustments on consequential grounds. For others, the intention is less than the deed; i.e., it permits one by a mental act to declare to be "unintended" the things one is going to do, thereby decreasing the dialogical credibility of one's justification.

Conceptual refinement has been disappointing; finally we turn to trace the problem of institutional credibility.

In the sociopolitical symbolism of public discourse, much is made of the control of the trigger by the national chief executive. The image of being constantly in charge is dramatized by a staff person constantly within reach carrying the codes needed to release retaliatory catastrophe. We are meant to believe that this dramatic scene-setting provides for a real decision which the chief executive would make under great pressure. Yet:

1. We cannot be sure how well the chief executive will be informed. How accurate will the kinds of data needed to enter into such a decision be?
2. The chief executive might make a decision on the basis of some proportionate judgment like "It is not worth exposing the United States to a massive retaliation just in order to save Würzburg from Soviet tanks." That would be to reject the first-strike escalation option, which, however, he or she believes is the reason for the threatening weapons buildup.
3. It may be that when pressed the president would act on the basis of a humane "stance" or "feel" like "Now that deterrence has failed, there is nothing to gain from killing two hundred million more." That would define our prior stance as having been "bluff" after all, though not premeditatedly so.
4. It is just as possible that the chief executive will be thrown into the "tragic macho" stance or feel, saying, "We will show them that we were

not bluffing," counter to any consequential rationality, to say nothing of morality. "Revenge" would be a euphemism for this; it would be gratuitous spasmic destruction.

5. If after all that buildup the president does say "no," would everyone in a silo or a sub with a finger on a nuclear trigger get the word? Obey it?

If the theatrical image of a real choice made by a chief executive under pressure in a few minutes is to be taken seriously, we need to be reassured that a "no" decision is a real possibility. The reality of that decision is indispensable if, in line with the theory of deterrence, we are to respect a distinction between threat and use. Yet:

1. There is serious doubt that such a distinction is possible in a democracy where the chief executive is (far more than a hereditary monarch or a dictator would be) a prisoner of the public postures and private deals whereby he or she came into office.
2. It is hard to make it credible in the face of institutional realism about the commitment of the professional military machinery to a spectrum of scenarios which, however variegated in detail otherwise, do not ever provide for surrender, do provide a high degree of field command autonomy in situations of communication collapse, and intentionally tend to erode the qualitative lines between kinds of weapons.

It may be that to acknowledge the failure of the model of sovereign decision making may lead us to a better picture of the shape of the deterrence issue. The many-factored diversity of dimensions in just-war reasoning makes it practically unavoidable that in the course of any one argument the weight shifts from one question to another, making it hard to pursue a single line of reasoning to some clear conclusion. Discussion about proportionality of damage shifts into debate about technological or political predictability. Discussion about innocence shifts into debate about whether in a democratic society one can distinguish between the government and the people. The particular shift that concerns us now has to do with the difficulty in knowing whose decision responsibility we are talking about when looking forward to the possible use—especially the possible extensive use—of nuclear weapons in the name of democratic governments.

The just-war tradition developed in a time of autocratic government.

If there was ever a morally accountable decision made about going to war, it was made by an individual. Whether that was a local baron or a national king, and whether he took counsel with his confessor or his cupbearer, his wife or his knights, one can still envisage the decision process as centered on one point in time and in the mind and will of one individual. One could work with the hypothetical model of "a decision," both with regard to the initiation of hostilities and concerning the choice of weapons. In our technological world this is not possible, even in societies having the outward appearance of dictatorship. Even the masters of the Kremlin need to juggle the forces of the military professionals, the economic producers, the secret police, the universities, the intellectuals, and the ethnic blocs. Even Somoza had to negotiate with businessmen and to resolve conflicts within his network of corruption. But what interests us now is not that technology makes the decision model incredible even in a dictatorship, but that democracy makes it categorically unthinkable.

Then the situation of a democracy, in which the person holding office has been chosen on the grounds of having most adequately won the moral support of a plurality of the electorate, does not provide the same leeway which an absolute monarch would have to digress from that community commitment either way, whether to be more respectful of the rights of others or to be less concerned for others and more concerned with simple self-interest. A leader elected by democratic process will thereby have promised to represent a particular interpretation of the national interest and identity. In times of major reorientation, this mandate may include dimensions of reform, review, or even repentance in the name of the nation, as for instance when the French elected Pierre Mendes-France to get them out of Vietnam. Very seldom, however, will there be exceptions to the general rule, long ago identified by Reinhold Niebuhr, to the effect that communities are generally less able to be unselfish than individuals, and that civilly structured communities are less able than voluntary ones. It will be rare that a bearer of elected political office will have a mandate to be rigorous about respecting just-war limitations. Far more easily, and in fact cheaply, a mandate can reflect national jingoism on the part of a fickle electorate. We observed how Ronald Reagan's standing went up after the internationally illegal attack on Granada, and Margaret Thatcher's after the disproportionate war in the South Atlantic.

Democracy does not therefore increase the potential for wise decisions.

Our concern is now specifically for wise choices in a situation of nuclear threat and counterthreat, coming on the tail of an escalation of subnuclear threats or attacks. The theory of deterrence says, if taken straight, that one may threaten to react to an enemy offense with a massive nuclear strike, but one may never do it. A dictator or medieval duke keeping his own counsel could possibly maintain that distinction between a threat and its effective execution, but it would seem that a democratically elected government cannot.

The current discussion, including the bishops' letter, seems quite unconcerned with identifying this question. The bishops do not enter into the discussion of who makes command decisions, thereby avoiding as well the complexities of decision-making prerogatives and capacities. Careful pastoral attention is given at the end of the letter to the challenge facing each of numerous categories of the flock: military professionals, young people, educators, people working in weapons industries, but never is the specific person responsible for the actual use of the weapons named. Only thanks to this gap were the drafters able to maintain an apparently strong statement that massive use would always be wrong, side by side with condoning deterrence through the threat of massive use for a time.

If there were more firm attention to the real institutional modalities of decision, the fact would then have to be faced that there is no middle ground between a real threat (i.e., a threat the adversary has strong reason to expect will be carried out) and an increasingly transparent bluff. The word *bluff* as was shown is not a fully appropriate phrase, since we know that the material means for the execution of the threat are at hand. What we do not know is whether moral or political restraints exist against its being carried out. Any observer of a society as permeated with humane values as is our own will know that an act of retaliation, pointless to prevent the attack for which it retaliates, adding destruction to destruction, would be unacceptable to many, and even to many who previously would have felt the deterrent posture to be unavoidable.

As intelligent social beings capable of imagining future decision settings, we already know that one cannot affirm in advance the moral legitimacy of a massive second strike under any probable circumstances. In an open society there is no way that that awareness can be kept from being returned to the precrisis thinking not only of political decision makers but also of the military commanders who are constantly preparing, under all sorts of discipline, for the time when they might be commanded to do the unthinkable. Since they are preparing not only mentally but institutionally to do it, it is not unthinkable. The entire credibility of the deterrent operation consists in the authenticity of their readiness to carry through with the threat precisely at the point where it would have become politically pointless and morally catastrophic.

The dilemma between readiness to go on with the immoral act, in order to make the deterrent credible ex post facto, and an empty threat, tempting the adversary to a test of luck, is not a debating maneuver of the nuclear pacifists. It is an internal paradox in the position of those who, like the bishops, seek to reject both a massive nuclear attack and the imperative of disarmament. It is not the kind of paradox whereby each component of an apparently contradictory set of ideas is more credible because the other stands in tension with it. It is rather a contradiction, whose unsustainable quality can only be hidden by patterns of reasoning that avoid facing the whole truth at the same time.

Believing as I do that ethics can and should be rational, methodologically self-aware, coherent, dialogical, and capable of transcending visceral intuitionism and arbitrariness by means of accountable language, I should be grateful if any discipline could be brought to the above problem by someone who would clarify the categories of "intention" or "threat"; but I have thus far seen no grounds to hold that it has been done, or even that clear progress is being made toward achieving it by the people who claim that the just-war tradition is morally credible.

Believing as I do that a gracious God can use inadequate instruments to help fallible people on the way to less inhumane ways of getting along together, I do not ask of any set of tools (neither of the just-war tradition as a whole, nor of double-effect reasoning, nor of metaethical or metalinguistic clarification) that it should function perfectly or without gaps. But I have not yet seen the tools that can keep the promise to stiffen moral judgment relatively.

Believing as I have for years that in the hands of *some* people *some* use of just-war categories can have both intellectual and institutional integrity, I am on the lookout for ways in which the just-war grid can motivate or undergird moral seriousness. I have seen some of these, but among contemporary ethicists, the ones who seem to me to do that with the most coherence are those who reject the deterrent threat, rather than those who seek to make room for it.

Notes

1. For a historical treatment of the just-war tradition, see James Turner Johnson, *Just-War Tradition and the Restraint of War: A Moral and Historical Inquiry* (Princeton: Princeton University Press, 1981).

2. John Cardinal Krol, "Testimony before the Senate Foreign Relations Committee, September 6, 1979," in Robert Heyer, ed., *Nuclear Disarmament: Key Statements of Popes, Bishops, Councils, and Churches* (New York: Paulist Press, 1982), 104.

3. See G. E. M. Anscombe, *Intention* (Ithaca, N.Y.: Cornell University Press, 1957). For further treatment of Anscombe's position, see Cora Diamond and Jenny Teichman, eds., *Intention and Intentionality: Essays in Honor of G. E. M. Anscombe* (Ithaca, N.Y.: Cornell University Press, 1979).

4. For Michael Novak's most extensive elaboration of his position on nuclear ethics, see his *Moral Clarity in the Nuclear Age* (Nashville, Tenn.: Thomas Nelson, 1983).

The Limits and Possibilities
of the New Technologies

5 • Deterrence, Defense, or War-Fighting? A Just-War Analysis of Some Recent Strategic Developments

JAMES TURNER JOHNSON

Introduction

Moral analysis of warfare is never done once and for all time, since the phenomenon of war itself never stands still for long. Weapons change, alliances among nations wax and wane, domestic political attitudes and material conditions may be transformed within the societies of prospective belligerents. It is one thing to apply moral analysis—itself far from an exact science—to a state of affairs that obtained in the past, so as to enter the debate, for example, over the justice or injustice of the strategic bombing campaigns of World War II. It is quite another thing to apply the same sort of moral analysis to the possibilities that war may—or may not—bring in a future that can never be glimpsed in its fullness from the present.

The purpose of this essay is to bring to bear on certain recent strategic developments in the East-West power relation a moral analysis rooted in the perspectives of just-war tradition. Specifically, I will comment critically on the present shape of U.S. nuclear strategy, then on two new strategic developments possessing the potential to change this current strategic posture decisively: the Strategic Defense Initiative (SDI) and research and development aimed toward producing fractional megatonnage nuclear weapons of extremely high accuracy.

The Just-War Concept

The term *just war* conveys somewhat different ideas to different people. As I employ this term, it refers to a broad moral tradition that has developed in Western culture as a result of the interaction of certain religious and secular forces, principally Christian theological ethics and canon law, secular law both domestic and international, the practice of relations among states, and the traditions of professional military life.

While the deepest roots of this tradition are to be found in the Hebraic and Greco-Roman antecedents to Western culture and in early Christian thought, we know it today substantially in the conceptual form that was given just-war doctrine in the late Middle Ages and the early modern period. In that form the concept of just war is developed under two rubrics, the *jus ad bellum,* having to do with when it is just to resort to arms, and the *jus in bello,* having to do with what limits ought to be observed in fighting justly. The former includes, maximally, seven ideas: that there must be just cause for resort to arms, that there must be due political authority for the decision to take arms, that the intention in doing so must be correct, that the good done by protection of values in this way must exceed the harm, that there must be a reasonable hope of success in the decision to take arms, that this decision must be a last resort, and that the end sought must be a renewed state of peace. The *jus in bello* includes two major ideas: that noncombatants should be spared direct, intentional harm, and that disproportionately destructive force should be avoided in the conduct of hostilities.[1]

The specific content assigned to each of these categories has varied somewhat over time and according to the context addressed by particular elements within the overall tradition. Thomas Aquinas in the thirteenth century, for example, identified three types of just cause: punishment of evil, repelling of an injury in progress (defense), and the need to recover something wrongly taken.[2] Just-war historian Alfred Vanderpol, commenting on Thomas's doctrine, argues that the punishment of evil was preeminent among these, and further that it remained the primary notion of just cause in church teaching throughout the Middle Ages.[3] By contrast, in twentieth-century international law the idea of defense is clearly the preeminent concept.[4] While it can be argued that the definition of defense can reasonably be stretched to include the other two ideas enumerated by Thomas,[5] the most striking development in twentieth-century thought on the justification of war is the extension of the category of defense to cover strategic nuclear retaliation. Whether deterrence by threat of retaliation is genuinely defense is a major moral issue raised by SDI, as we shall see below.

Alongside such particular changes as the concept of just cause there has been something of a sea change within the *jus ad bellum* of just-war tradition as a whole. While medieval and early modern theorists treated the categories of just cause, right authority, and right intention as more important than the other *jus ad bellum* ideas, contemporary moral concerns have tended to stress precisely those concepts paid little attention by these earlier theorists: proportionality, last resort, and the restoration of peaceful relations in the international community. While this implicit prioritization of the *jus ad bellum* ideas can be found in major ecclesiastical position statements (notably the argument of the U.S. Catholic bishops in their 1983 pastoral letter, *The Challenge of Peace*),[6] the principal reason for the shift of emphasis lies in the nature of modern international law, which has constituted a major vehicle for development of just-war thought and practice since the time of Grotius. In the international law redaction of just-war tradition the existence of sovereign political entities is taken for granted, and there is no attempt to judge the rightness or wrongness of the governing authority of any particular one of them. Right authority thus becomes the *competence de guerre* enjoyed by the ruling person or body of any independent state. Just cause devolves into defense against attack—narrowly understood as firing the second shot in response to the first shot already fired by an attacker—and right intention thus is defined implicitly as that of defending against attack. With the exception of the definition of just cause in terms of defense, international law pays little or no attention to these *jus ad bellum* categories. By contrast, international law has a major interest in maintaining the status quo of relations among nations, and this leads to greater attention to the effort to minimize or eliminate any resort to armed force (the just-war concept of last resort) found in the League of Nations Covenant, the establishment of the World Court, the Pact of Paris, and the United Nations Charter. The just-war category of the end of peace, redefined as the restoration of a tolerable stability among nations without use of armed force, follows from the same concerns. The stress on considerations of proportionality—counting the likely overall costs of an armed conflict and weighing them against the goods to be defended—has been in large part a result of reflection on the destructiveness of modern war and, particularly since 1945, of nuclear war.[7]

In the *jus in bello* the concepts of noncombatant protection and proportionality in the sense of matching level of force employed to the desired goal have, in general, risen in importance relative to the *jus ad bellum* over time. Some contemporary critics of military preparedness have argued that war today is inherently unjust because it can never meet these *jus in bello* criteria.[8] This is in sharp contrast to the main line of just-war tradition, even today, which regards these *jus in bello* criteria as coming into play only after the initial decision has been made that a resort to armed conflict is justified.[9] Certainly it is necessary to say that moral consideration of whether a prospective use of armed force will be just requires taking account of *jus in bello* concerns; this is not the same, though, as saying that the latter should dominate or overrule the former.

Where do we stand—or ought we to stand—today relative to this tradition on the justification and limitation of war? It must be said first that for the main line of Western culture, there is really no getting away from either the conceptual categories of just-war thought or, I think, the main line of the content of these categories as this has consensually developed over the centuries. While some critical voices contend today that just-war thinking is irrelevant to the nuclear age, the fact is that the concepts and content of this tradition are so tightly interwoven with Western moral and political concepts and institutions as a whole that we could not reject this one part of the whole fabric without calling in question the rest as well. James Childress, addressing this character of the just-war categories, argues that they are experienced as imposing prima facie duties on us.[10] I would go further: these categories, originating as they have in the communal experience of Western culture over centuries, express fundamental values that lie near the core of the moral identity of this culture. When we say that there should be a just cause for resort to armed force, this is a way of saying that coercion by armed force is not morally neutral but needs to be justified by some grave reason; when we say that the resort to force should be a last resort and should be aimed at producing peace, this is a way of expressing a bias toward peace instead of war and toward the solution of disputes by nonmilitary means where possible; when we say that harm to noncombatants should be avoided, this is an affirmation of the idea that people who do not themselves directly cause harm should not have harm directed at them; and so on for all of the nine major analytical categories or criteria of just-war tradition.

Just-war tradition is not, contrary to much popular usage, a doctrine. Rather it is the result of the combination of many doctrines from various theoretical and existential perspectives over a history many centuries long. The proper use of this tradition for moral guidance requires entering the circle of witnesses provided by this history, taking seriously both what they agree upon in common and the elements of difference or tension among them, along with the reasons for such difference. In this way the debates of the past can be brought to bear on the debates of the present.

A Critique of Nuclear Deterrence Strategy

The strategy of nuclear deterrence is often represented as a means of defense, but it is more properly described as an effort to deter attack by threatening unacceptable damage in retaliation for such attack. Defense, as understood in just-war tradition and in military and political parlance prior to the nuclear age, referred to measures designed to prevent an attack from succeeding. A strategy of defense, then, in this sense, would be one of denial of victory to the attacker. Such a strategy defines force structures, types of weapons, and deployment patterns designed to be used against enemy forces deployed against them, and it implies military research and development oriented toward improving such "war-fighting" capacity. Such a strategy also has a deterrent aspect, however, along with its war-fighting thrust: no prospective enemy, when counting costs and measuring the likelihood of success, could be expected rationally to set an armed conflict in motion knowing that success was unlikely or that the costs of success would be unacceptably high.

In any case, nuclear deterrence strategy in the broad form it has taken over the past forty years is a strategy of retaliation, not of defense; it aims at punishing the enemy for harm already given, not at warding off the harm as it is being dealt out and preventing its effects from being felt on the values of the society being defended. The difference can be seen in the simple realization that, should deterrence by threat of unacceptable punishment fail and a nuclear attack be launched, no amount of after-the-fact retaliation would prevent severe damage to the society or societies to be defended and forfeiture of values that were ostensibly protected by the retaliatory threat. A strategy of defense by victory-denial, however, still may operate to protect such societies and their values even after deterrence breaks down and armed conflict begins.

The argument is often made that nuclear retaliation strategy has been dictated by the nature of the technology of nuclear weapons. On this widely popular argument there could be no other strategy than one based on threat of retaliation for use of nuclear weapons and for protection against their use on Western societies. This is, however, an oversimplification that overlooks the major values assumptions that have also affected the shape of strategic nuclear doctrine. Concepts of nuclear weapons and their use have evolved in U.S. doctrine in a direct line from the concepts associated with strategic bombing in World War II. The acceptance of countercity bombing in this war rested, in turn, on the experience of countercity bombardment during World War I. Admittedly, in all these cases technology was a significant factor: for example, the inability of weapons delivery systems to discriminate closely enough to allow avoidance of harm to noncombatants even if desired. But an important shift in values also occurred which was not itself driven by technology. This was an erosion of the moral ideal of protecting noncombatants so far as possible. In the World War II debates over strategic bombing this erosion of the ideal of noncombatant immunity appeared in the idea that all citizens of the enemy state were one's enemies, and that it was a proper act of war to attack the military capabilities of troops in line of battle by attacking the morale of civilians at home. This shift in moral values was symbolized by the new concept of "the home front" alongside the old one of "the battlefront."[11]

Strategic nuclear retaliatory doctrine, then, as it developed after World War II, carried forward tendencies and assumptions already shaped in that war and earlier, and it rests on a mix that includes ideological as well as technological factors. Rather than the one driving the other, there has been a mutual interaction of the two. The decision to use the original atomic bombs against cities in which civilian and military elements were mixed was preceded and influenced by a history of conventional countercity bombing; it was the perceived lack of moral problem with such bombing that made such use of the atomic bombs seem right, not the technology of the bombs or their delivery systems. (Indeed, the first delivery systems were the same manned bombers that had been used for strategic bombing with conventional high explosives. Only the form of the explosive was different, and the convention of measuring the destructive capability of nuclear weapons in terms of equivalent tonnage of TNT shows the desire, in strategic terms, to assimilate the new forms of weaponry to the old.) Later in the nuclear age, a similar value orientation led to the development of fusion warheads of massive destructive power. The combined technological factors of the destructiveness of these warheads and the inaccuracy of early ballistic delivery systems meant that the only reasonable strategy that could have been developed around them was a countercity one; yet the moral decision that it was justified to target population centers was an independent one that had already been made in earlier contexts.[12]

In just-war terms, the direct, intentional targeting of noncombatants is immoral. This fact informs contemporary just-war theorizing in a variety of ways. Paul Ramsey, in books published in 1961 and 1968,[13] argued that while direct, intentional targeting of noncombatants is morally wrong, this is not the same as saying that any harm to noncombatants in a war renders the war unjust. Rather, Ramsey reasoned by use of the moral rule of double effect, if the actual target (say, a military base or a missile site) is legitimate, then indirect, unintentional harm to noncombatants may be allowed, though there is still an obligation to avoid such harm where possible. This line of reasoning has an obvious force, though it eventually runs into difficulty: when scores of multimegatonnage nuclear warheads are targeted on legitimate military objectives in and around a particular population center,[14] common sense cannot discriminate between the intention to attack those legitimate objectives directly and the intention to attack the densely packed noncombatant population in the surrounding area. Indeed, in such a context an appeal to the rule of double effect to justify such targeting may be indistinguishable from mere ratiocination. Use of the rule of double effect in the context of targeting of massively destructive warheads delivered on military targets in the midst of population centers does not satisfy just-war concerns for the protection of noncombatants.

In their 1983 pastoral letter the U.S. Catholic bishops recognized the immorality of direct, intentional attacks on noncombatants and expressed skepticism that use of strategic nuclear weapons would not violate noncombatant immunity; yet their attempt to resolve the moral issue was far from satisfactory. *The Challenge of Peace* distinguished between deterrence by *threat* of nuclear retaliation and actual *use* of strategic nuclear weapons. Such a threat, the bishops reasoned, is morally acceptable, though carrying out the threat by an actual counterpopulation strike would be morally wrong.[15] This rather ingenious bit of rationalization has already been the object of much debate. I have never found it the least bit persuasive, either as a moral argument or as a base for sound strategic thinking. Morally speaking, it is far from convincing to argue that it is acceptable to threaten to blow up another's house (along with his entire family and his next-door neighbors) as a means to keep him from blowing up your own. This is an immoral threat whether you actually intend to do what you threaten or possess the capability to do so. Yet the threat would not be credible were the capability to do so not in place; thus the dependence on the threat requires the existence of the capability to do what is threatened. In the case of strategic nuclear weapons, that capability implies the actual deployment and targeting of ballistic missiles.

The U.S. bishops were right to argue that, on the theoretical level, there is a moral distinction between the threat to use these missiles and the actual use of them: it is the distinction between a lesser and a greater evil. This *theoretical* distinction, though, does not translate into an *actual* difference on the level of practical morality and concrete deterrence strategy. A nuclear strategy based on the threat to retaliate without the capability to carry through on that threat and the embodied intention to do so would not long remain credible. To attempt to redefine the moral issue by separation of threat from use does not, then, resolve the moral problems inherent in use of nuclear weapons of the current strategic types. Indeed, if anything, it draws attention all the more sharply to these moral problems.

The current strategy of deterrence is in fact, as I argued above, a strategy based on the credible threat of retaliatory punishment. In just-war terms there is nothing inherently immoral about a strategy of punishment, despite the modern trend toward a moral rhetoric representing the only just cause for use of armed force to be defense. What determines whether it is wrong is the nature of the punishment and who receives it. Given a strategy that rests, today as in the past, on multimegaton nuclear warheads and a targeting doctrine that accepts multiple strikes on military targets inside centers of noncombatant population, neither appeal to the rule of double effect nor the effort to separate the deterrent threat from the retaliatory action itself can overcome the immorality inherent in such a strategy.

I argued earlier that the main line of nuclear strategy was driven by value assumptions as well as by the technology of nuclear weapons and delivery systems. Had the force of the moral ideal of noncombatant immunity not already eroded before the advent of the nuclear age, I doubt whether it would have seemed so right or so inevitable that nuclear weapons and nuclear strategy should have developed as they have. Similarly, if that moral ideal is now to be recovered and reasserted, this must imply changes in the nature of strategic doctrine and targeting policy, and in the weapons of defense and deterrence themselves.

Other moral concerns from just-war tradition also point toward the need to make such changes. Current strategic doctrine and weaponry do not, as noted above, provide a *defense* of values against an attack in progress but are suited only to *deter* attack. Ironically, carrying through the threatened punishment might, under some circumstances, itself serve to complete the destruction of the values ostensibly being preserved and protected. (This would be the case, for example, in a scenario in which a Soviet first strike was beneath the level necessary to produce a nuclear winter, while the addition of U.S. retaliatory strike would exceed this level.) Again, though it is always difficult to quantify good and evil, the magnitude of destruction that could be reasonably expected from a strategic nuclear exchange calls into question whether a war fought in this way could ever not cause a disproportion of bad over good. Nuclear pacifists, though they typically deride just-war theory as irrelevant to the nuclear age, have regularly argued their position in terms of this just-war criterion. Mennonite theologian John Howard Yoder, for example, has argued explicitly that faced with adding disproportionate harm to disproportionate harm, the more moral course for Americans in the event of a nuclear war would be simply to surrender.[16]

We may put the matter more positively by turning the critical focus of just-war tradition around to ask what sort of strategic posture is compatible with the moral concerns found here. In the first place, a bias toward defense rather than offense runs through just-war tradition as a whole, and it is especially strong, as noted earlier, in modern international law. Taken seriously, this implies development of weapons that are capable of providing genuine defense against attack, not only retaliatory punishment for attack. Second, there is a bias toward weaponry that is inherently not disproportionately destructive and is capable of being used discriminately against legitimate military targets.[17] This implies lowering the destructive capability of nuclear weapons, replacing at least some nuclear weapons with conventional ones, and increasing the accuracy and controllability of delivery systems.

In the following sections I will apply these standards of measurement to two new strategic developments, the Strategic Defense Initiative and fractional-megatonnage, high-accuracy strategic nuclear weapons.

The Case of SDI

The Strategic Defense Initiative has emerged as a central issue of disagreement between the United States and the Soviet Union in the arms control arena. This is not necessarily the most important thing to say about it, however, from a moral perspective based in just-war tradition. Arms control as such, as this is currently understood to mean limits on numbers and types of weapons, particularly strategic weapons, is not an end in itself, from a perspective within this tradition; it is, rather, at best a means to ends that are themselves morally justifiable.

Focusing on ends, not means, also shifts the debate over laboratory research versus testing versus deployment into a perspective different from that of the arms controllers. If strategic defense is itself morally justifiable, or justifiable in some forms but not in others, then all levels of work from research to deployment are justified. If the judgment is reached that strategic defense weapons systems, or some such weapons, are morally unjust, then earlier stages of work—and in particular, laboratory research—may still be justified if there is the possibility of producing moral benefits. Since most of the public debate has been carried on in terms of the narrow perspectives of arms control, these broader and more fundamental moral concerns have been largely disregarded.

Moral analysis of SDI is complicated by two further factors. First, attempts at moral justification have been a part of the SDI debate, on both sides, since its inception. Thus a just-war analysis will inevitably look, at times, like an effort to take sides in the debate that is already under way, rather than a fresh attempt to evaluate SDI in moral terms. Nonetheless, it is important to conduct such a just-war analysis, for doing so, along with providing a vehicle for judging SDI, also implicitly provides a perspective from which to judge the ostensibly moral claims that have already been advanced regarding this program.

A second complicating factor is the question of exactly what the term *SDI* means. President Reagan's initial rhetoric, in his address of March 23, 1983, seemed to hold out the promise of a defensive shield capable of protecting U.S. citizenry as a whole. Advertisements in support of SDI aired on U.S. television for a time in 1985 reinforced this image, employing a voice-over technique while on the screen appeared a drawing like a young child's in which a rainbowlike shield protected a house against incoming missiles. The actual shape of authorized SDI planning, though, so far as this can be made out from unclassified materials and public statements of military and administration spokespersons qualified to speak on SDI, is much more selective: for technical and economic reasons current planning is focused on the possibilities held out by SDI for reinforcing the survivability of the U.S. strategic retaliatory force.[18]

These are not necessarily contradictory concepts. One way of arguing for their complementarity is to describe the narrower version of SDI as the short-term goal, an initial step toward the implementation of the broader vision. Since admittedly the SDI program will be very expensive to bring to the deployment stage, and since it is dependent on extremely complex technology some of which is now only in the experimental stage, on this argument the proper first step is not to attempt to implement the broader counterpopulation shield in the first generation of space-based strategic defenses but to reserve that goal for subsequent generations of such defense systems. In this argument the high moral goal of counterpopulation defense is implicitly honored, but its realization is postponed for technological and economic reasons. A familiar operative rule of moral analysis is that no one is morally obligated to do something that is beyond his or her power; that rule is implicitly observed in this argument.

A second type of argument for the complementarity of the broader and narrower concepts of SDI is somewhat more complex, and it sharply shifts the ground of the moral reasoning regarding SDI. This argument is that the narrower version of SDI is valuable as an enhancement of strategic deterrence by threat of retaliatory punishment. By increasing the survivability of the U.S. land-based strategic nuclear force, SDI would reduce the possibility of a Soviet first strike, since that strike would be less punishing and a heavy retaliatory blow thus much more likely. We should recognize that this is a rather different kind of argument from the first one and is in tension with it. The first argument accepts the ideal of counterpopulation strategic defense, and a counterforce shield is understood as a first step toward that goal. The second, like all of the main line of deterrence strategy throughout its forty-year history, focuses not on counterpopulation defense against an attack in progress but rather on preventing such an attack from occurring in the first place by increasing the credibility of the threat of an unacceptably destructive retaliatory strike.

What of the connection between the narrower and broader defensive shields, according to this second argument? The answer, simply put, is that the concept of a full protective population shield is jettisoned. Population protection, on this argument, depends on the continuation of credible deterrence, and that rests on a retaliatory threat. Given an initial limited SDI capability to protect the strategic retaliatory force, a later broadening of SDI capability would still be first of all for the purpose of enhancing such protection. Some degree of increased population defense might well be a result of such a more capable system, but it would be a secondary result from the steps taken to reach the primary goal.

In short, the two lines of argument for SDI that I have sketched, together with their implications, lead squarely into a debate of long standing over the merits of defense as opposed to those of deterrence. Arguments opposed to SDI also lead toward this debate, though principally by one path only: the path that assumes the validity of deterrence doctrine and discounts the ideal of population defense.

War avoidance is certainly a major theme in just-war tradition, and it is the fundamental purpose embodied in the structure of strategic deterrence by threat of retaliation. What is morally problematic about this form of strategic deterrence is its failure to deal constructively with the eventuality that it might, under some conditions, fail to prevent a war from starting. In that eventuality it is reasonable to expect that the strategic nuclear weapons possessed by both sides would be used, with major destructive effect on noncombatants (including citizens of nonbelligerent states) even in the case of the most scrupulously discriminating choice of targets. The moral dilemma posed by reliance on strategic deterrence by threat of retaliation is that in case of the failure of deterrence to avoid war, the resulting conflict would likely be all the more destructive because of the use of the very weapons—strategic nuclear missiles—that were never supposed to have to be used.

So-called war-fighting planning is, by contrast, weakest in terms of its ability to avoid war altogether and strongest in its purpose of continuing to defend threatened values in the midst of an armed conflict. There is an important deterrent or war-avoiding element to such a strategic configuration, though its effect is generally downplayed by its critics; the aim here is deterrence by threat of denial of victory.

Moral and strategic concerns tend to converge, then, on the problem of the optimum mix in defense planning of war-avoidance (deterrence) and war-fighting (active defense of values). Strategic defense offers new possibilities in both these regards. Its actual capabilities remain unproved, and other means to optimizing these twin concerns may prove better, but it is worthwhile nonetheless to examine SDI in this light.

The major claimed benefit for the more limited form of strategic deterrence is that it would improve the survivability of U.S. land-based ICBMs, currently vulnerable to a first strike.[19] Not only would this in principle enhance the aim of war-avoidance, but since the weapons that would be protected include precisely those that would be most capable of being used in accord with the just-war principles of discrimination (noncombatant immunity) and proportion, this would be a positive development in *jus in bello* terms as well.

On the negative side, it has been argued by critics of SDI that it would be provocative and destabilizing. A *New York Times* article, "Dark Side of 'Star Wars': System Could Also Attack,"[20] summarizes some critics' fears about the offensive capability of space-based lasers: they might be used to "deliver devastating non-nuclear strikes to high-value targets anywhere on the earth's surface, in the air or in space, . . . with no collateral damage to adjacent civilian populations." "Key targets" might include oil tankers at sea, petroleum storage depots on land, power transformers, military vehicles, troops, and even grain fields and storage bins. A much more recent article[21] states that, for technical reasons, "space-based lasers . . . have been abandoned," and if true this renders the above argument against SDI moot. Nonetheless, we should dwell a moment on the language of the critic quoted. From a just-war perspective it would be a decided *advantage,* not a disadvantage, to be able to deliver nonnuclear strikes against legitimate military targets without collateral damage to adjacent civilian populations. Given that today's nuclear missiles can destroy high-value targets anywhere on the globe but at the cost of such collateral damage, a space-based laser would be a much more morally defensible weapon in terms of the ideals of discrimination and proportionality.

The most significant benefits, indeed, potentially offered by SDI lie in the region of war-fighting means and methods, the arena of the just-war *jus in bello.* If there was ever a weapon inherently offensive in character, it is the multimegaton nuclear warhead. While there are certainly offensive possibilities for the more exotic new technologies being researched for SDI—notably lasers and particle beams—these possibilities could scarcely pose worse problems than those of strategic nuclear weapons now deployed. Less exotic technologies—for example, the use of antimissile missiles and "smart rocks"—pose no inherent offensive threat; they are purely defensive by their nature.

For just-war tradition, though, the most fundamental issues in the war-fighting context are defined by the moral criteria of discrimination and proportionality. These criteria imply the development and deployment of weapons that are highly accurate, limited in their collateral effects, and maximally subject to human control.

Applying these guidelines to particular weapons or weapons systems requires comparing them with rival weapons or systems, and it requires setting them in the context of their strategic and tactical purpose. Thus, for example, compared with the tactical fission warheads that they replaced, and in the strategic and tactical context of their intended use, the miniaturized fusion ("enhanced radiation" or "neutron") warheads now deployed in NATO forces are morally superior because of their lessened collateral damage due to blast and long-lived radiation effects. Since conventional weapons able to perform the same functions would likely cause far more blast and fire damage than the enhanced radiation warheads, there may even be an edge in favor of the latter here. Similarly, a high-accuracy (low-CEP) ballistic or cruise missile is morally superior to one less accurate because it can, in principle, be used more discriminatingly (that is, so as better to avoid collateral noncombatant harm from a strike against a combatant target). Moreover, since for effectiveness against a given target the size of the warhead can decrease as accuracy increases, the low-CEP weapon may also be more able to satisfy the moral requirement of proportionality.[22]

Measured against strategic nuclear weapons, the systems that are projected as part of SDI more closely conform to the criteria of discrimination and proportionality. They are to be counterforce weapons by design, and their collateral effect on noncombatants when used in this manner would, so far as can be told, be nil. Even if they were used in a counterpopulation mode, as the critic quoted earlier has suggested they might be, the effects of a thermonuclear explosion would be far less discriminate and far more disproportionately destructive of noncombatant lives and values.

These reflections apply to both the narrower and the broader conceptions of strategic defense as defined earlier. It is not necessary to imagine a defensive screen over the whole of U.S. society—difficult or impossible to achieve by current technology or that projected for the next decade—to recognize that, in terms of the categories of just-war tradition, strategic defense is morally superior to a continued reliance on strategic nuclear deterrence as the main line of the West's effort to protect and preserve its values.

Improvements in Nuclear Missiles

Moral responsibility does not end when a war begins. Rather, with the onset of armed conflict a new dimension to that responsibility opens up: the need to fight so as to effectively protect and preserve the values being fought for without using methods and means that would themselves call those values into question. The *jus in bello* of just-war tradition, in coalescing around the importance of avoiding harm to noncombatants and limiting the destructiveness of means of force employed, itself is a statement of value.

The principle of noncombatant immunity is a particular crystallization of the more fundamental moral conception that it is not right to harm the innocent. This principle is, for the *jus in bello,* what the idea of just cause is for the *jus ad bellum.* Those who may be opposed by force are thus those who themselves are doing wrong by force. Combatants do such wrong; noncombatants do not. Whatever their own sympathies may be assumed to be, then, the noncombatant population of an enemy state in wartime do not give up their moral status unless they themselves take up arms or move into positions of close support to those who actually bear arms. It is sometimes claimed that in modern war there are no noncombatants. This may be simply the argument that attitudes, not actions, make enemies, and that in a modern state it may be assumed that the civilian population wants their nation to win in war, just as do the soldiers in arms. Yet the antipathetic attitude of others does not in itself justify using armed force against them, much less killing them.[23] Or the argument that in modern war there are no noncombatants may be based on the alleged close ties to the civilian and military sectors in modern economies. The worker at a plant that makes ball bearings used in tanks does not himself bear arms, but he is nonetheless directly aiding the war effort. The answer to this line of argument is, of course, different depending on the type of example given. Yet even if the worker in question is a combatant, his bedridden father at home is not, nor his wife who has small children at home, nor those children. Broadening the category of combatants to include people in civilian clothes and civilian jobs like that of the ball-bearing worker does not do away with the fact that, in a modern society as well as in any in the past, there remain some persons and classes of persons who are genuinely noncombatants, to whom is owed a moral duty not to give direct and intentional harm.

The *jus in bello* principle of proportionality also echoes the moral concerns encapsulated in the *jus ad bellum*. This principle reminds us that the justification of use of armed force does not extend to the infliction of gratuitous destruction or the establishment of a Carthaginian peace. This just-war concept does not mean, as is sometimes argued, opposing force with like or equal force to produce a stalemate; nor does it imply only defensive configurations and use of military force.[24] Rather it means simply that if a particular military objective is justified, then the force employed to attain it should be the minimum consistent with that object. Anything more is gratuitous.

Both these moral principles from the just-war *jus in bello* point in the same direction. Weapons of war should be, by design, highly controllable and relatively limited in their destructive effects. For noncombatant immunity, controllability means the ability to discriminate between legitimate targets and noncombatants in the immediate area, while limitation of destructiveness means both minimizing the collateral deaths and damage that will occur around the target and also minimizing the long-term effects of the damage that will linger after the end of the war, when all are noncombatants. For proportionality, controllability means the ability to match countermeasures more precisely to threats, and limited destructiveness means the ability to neutralize a threat without gratuitous destruction to nearby values it would be well to preserve.

The above considerations are not new; Paul Ramsey advanced very similar arguments in his first book on nuclear war, published in 1961, reasoning from them to the moral preferability of counterforce over counterpopulation (countervalue) targeting of nuclear weapons.[25] When the actual weapons that might be targeted in a counterforce mode are considered, however, it quickly becomes apparent that, for multimegaton warheads, even if delivered by vehicles with a reasonable accuracy, in practical terms there will be no difference between targeting a military installation in the center of a concentration of noncombatant population and targeting that noncombatant population itself. If we wish to take seriously such a realization while maintaining a commitment to the moral ideals of proportionality and noncombatant immunity, there are but a few alternative ways to do so.

1. We may identify nuclear weapons as a class with indiscriminate and disproportionate destruction and decide that therefore no circumstances exist in which they could be used morally. Taken in one direction, this path

leads to total nuclear disarmement. Taken another way, it leads to the position of the U.S. Catholic bishops that deterrence by threat of nuclear retaliation is morally permissible, but the retaliation that is threatened would not be moral to carry out. Lacking such general disarmament and recognizing the implausibility that threat and use can be separated as the U.S. bishops desired, this way of dealing with the moral issue leaves a great deal wanting.

2. We may argue, as Ramsey did in 1961, that the important moral concern is to avoid direct, intentional attacks on noncombatants. Ramsey employed the rule of double effect to argue that where harm to non-combatants is an indirect, unintended secondary effect of a legitimate military action, then it is excused. This makes another distinction, like that between threat and use made by the U.S. Catholic bishops, that is more persuasive in theoretical than in practical context. Though military and combatant civilian installations in or near a given city may be the direct targets, for the case of multimegaton weapons it is implausible to separate the intention of crippling these targets from that of harming the noncombatant population in the immediate vicinity. Where the area of destruction extends out from the point of detonation to include a hundred square miles or more, to call that destruction "secondary" and "unin-tended" is to twist the meanings of those words beyond reason.

3. We may decide to limit our use of such weapons to targets in un-populated or sparsely populated areas, such as a naval battle group at sea or missile silos located in remote areas. In moral terms this would be about the limit of appropriate use of very large nuclear weapons, and a targeting plan for such weapons should at the very least give priority to this concept. Yet such targeting alone would be a severe restriction on the actual use of nuclear weapons, and it is not likely that without expansion of the target list beyond the bounds of discrimination and proportionality this could provide either a workable deterrence or a workable war-fighting plan. As one critic of strategic nuclear weapons has argued, "If you take the cities out of the war-plan, there's no war-plan left."[26]

4. We might choose to accelerate development and deployment of alternative types of weapons able to replace those that are by design inca-pable of being used against most legitimate targets without being indis-criminate and disproportionate. This would include delivery systems of very low CEP mated to either fractional megatonnage nuclear warheads or conventional high-explosive warheads. Since research and develop-

ment, and some deployment, of such systems has already been under way for some time, the decision to seek the solution to the moral dilemma of how to protect values worth defending by just means is not just an expression of an ideal; it is rather the choice of an option for both deterrence and possible war-fighting that at once draws us closer to the goals of discrimination and proportion in our use of military force and to what is actually possible in weapons technology and force configurations built around it.

Counterforce targeting is, in short, implied by just-war concerns. Yet without means capable of being employed against forces without indiscriminate and disproportionate collateral harm to values, adoption of the counterforce ideal remains empty of real content and, at bottom, a moral sham. Weaponry capable of being used in a counterforce mode without such indiscriminate and disproportionate effects, together with strategy and tactics that maximize the ability of such weaponry to keep the use of military force within these moral limits, is a direct implication of taking seriously the requirements of the *jus in bello* of just-war tradition.

Now, how does reality—what is currently the case and what is reasonably expected to be possible in the near future—fit with this moral goal? Unlike the case of SDI, where most of the technology is still in the stage of research and much of it is new and untried, the move toward low-CEP delivery vehicles and fractional megatonnage nuclear warheads is already well under way in Western forces. The U.S. Minuteman III with Mk-12A reentry vehicle has a CEP of approximately .10 nautical miles (or 200 meters) and a warhead whose yield is .335 megatons. Such a warhead is still too destructive to be usable, following just-war standards, against targets in or near centers of noncombatant population. For such use both CEP and warhead yield would have to be reduced still further. The Pershing II has achieved a CEP of .015 nautical miles (30 meters), and the technology appears available to reduce CEP still further to the range of .005 nautical miles (or 10 meters). Lowering the yield of nuclear warheads to the range of .5 kiloton (.0005 megaton) is also possible.[27] Such a warhead would be vastly less destructive than the current Minuteman III warhead mentioned above and another quantum leap away from the destructiveness of the multimegaton warheads now deployed by both the United States and the Soviet Union. (The largest warhead now deployed is Soviet, with a yield of 20 megatons. Such a weapon is essentially a counterpopulation weapon, whatever the ostensible targeting.) Now, .5 kiloton is the equivalent of 500 pounds of high explosives, and this has been one of the standard sizes of high-explosive bombs since World War II. In other words, when this range is reached—and indeed, considerably before it, if the comparison is between multiple conventional weapons and one nuclear warhead—there is a real option of substituting non-nuclear for nuclear warheads, given delivery vehicles of sufficient carrying capacity.

Another factor is whether the intended target is "hard" or "soft." Counter-*nuclear*-force targeting must assume "hard" targets, that is, reinforced concrete missile silos. Against such targets the CEP-yield ratio is crucial, for what matters is producing the blast pressure necessary to fracture the silo and render its missile inoperable. High-CEP weapons thus correlate with high yields and use of multiple warheads per target. (CEP, after all, is a measure of *probable* error, and a given missile may fall outside the average CEP radius, where it will fail to achieve the desired effect.)

Replacement of low-accuracy (high-CEP), high-yield weapons with newer types of high accuracy and commensurately lower yield has benefits in terms of the *jus in bello* concepts even when the target is in a remote area. After the Chernobyl disaster it is absurd to minimize the effect of nuclear fallout on populations even hundreds of miles away. Similarly, the atmospheric detonation of a high-yield strategic nuclear warhead, even if used in a counterforce mode against a remotely located silo, will inevitably produce counterpopulation effects in the form of radioactive fallout in areas far removed from the target silo. In the real world of nuclear strategy we must magnify these effects by two (since typically two warheads are assigned to each hard target), multiply by the number of hard targets, then add the number of soft targets against which a single warhead will suffice. The result is massive noncombatant devastation, which is immoral even if we do not go so far as to postulate nuclear winter or, in Jonathan Schell's terms, "a republic of insects and grass."[28]

By contrast, increasing accuracy of delivery vehicles (lowering the CEP) allows lowering the yield of the warhead, since the desired blast pressure against hard targets can be had with lower yield when the placement of the warhead is more precise. The increase in accuracy may also make it possible to use only one, not two, warheads per hard target. Using a CEP of .015 nautical miles and a desired blast pressure of 5000 pounds per square inch, but still assuming two warheads per hard target, a recent article puts the necessary yield at 1.2 kilotons (.0012 megatons) for each such target.[29] Again, here we are in the range of conventional high explosives. Yet even without substituting high-explosive warheads for nuclear ones, there is a vast difference between the collateral harm caused by a nuclear explosion of .0012 megatons and one of .670 megatons (that is, two of the U.S. Mk-12A warheads mentioned above), let alone one of 40 megatons (two of the 20-megaton Soviet warheads mentioned above). Even if we do not assume that targets in or near noncombatant population centers are among those chosen for actual destruction, there is a clear imperative, for persons concerned with the moral right of noncombatants to protection in war, to develop counterforce weaponry that will produce the lowest yield possible, thus producing the lowest collateral harm to noncombatants consistent with destruction of the legitimate targets.

Conclusion

Just-war thinking remains relevant in the contemporary world. It could hardly be done away with in any case, because it is part of the cultural heritage of the West and expresses a long-term historical consensus on when values should be protected by force and what kinds of force are appropriate for the protection of value. In other words, this tradition tells us something of who we are and what we hold dear, and without it our culture would be different in ways difficult to imagine. But more than this, the tradition holds implications for present moral analysis and decisions affecting the future which we would be ill-advised to ignore. Contemporary military analysis is full to the brim with unidimensional arguments. The arms control community attempts to reduce everything to what helps or hinders arms control; members of the deterrence community focus on what is perceived by them as creating greater deterrent stability or impairing that stability; nuclear pacifists hate weapons of any kind as such and value disarmament at whatever cost; extreme hawks work for overkill capability whatever the results that might follow in case of war. So often in recent debate the issues have been stated in terms of the value of deterrence over defense, the value of second-strike weapons (by definition too low in accuracy to be useful in a first strike, but also high in yield as a result of their CEP) over those that could be useful in a first strike. Just-war tradition helps to return the moral debate to fundamentals: there may be expected to be occasions in which the only way to protect the values we hold dear is by use of military force, and it is justified to seek to protect these values by force in such cases; yet not any and all kinds of military force may morally be employed, since some would result in destroying those values themselves. Defense of values, not offensive endangerment of the values of others, is a bias in just-war tradition. Avoidance of harm to noncombatants and of disproportionate, gratuitous destruction is also a bias within this tradition. The tradition further serves as a reminder that we live in a world in which the end of all war—all threat to value by force—is not a reality, so that it is wrong to pretend that it is. It reminds us, finally, that we must make concrete judgments regarding weapons, strategies, and tactics to seek to optimize the goods we seek to preserve. I have argued that just-war considerations tend to produce a positive assessment of SDI and that they very definitely point to adoption of low-CEP, fractional megatonnage nuclear weapons. Neither of these is good in itself; yet, in the real world of human history we must compare them with the strategies and weaponry of nuclear deterrence as it has existed previously. The moral choices reached from this perspective will not look attractive to many persons whose prior commitments lock them within narrower points of view. Nor will the relativity of the moral choices implied by just-war considerations be attractive to persons gripped by a utopian vision of a world in which there is no violence. The contemporary relevance of just-war tradition nevertheless perseveres.

Notes

1. For more on these categories and their historical development see my *Ideology, Reason, and the Limitation of War* (Princeton: Princeton University Press, 1975) and *Just War Tradition and the Restraint of War* (Princeton: Princeton University Press, 1981); Frederick H. Russell, *The Just War in the Middle Ages* (Cambridge: Cambridge University Press, 1975); William V. O'Brien, *The Conduct of Just and Limited War* (New York: Praeger Publishers, 1981); and Paul Ramsey, *War and the Christian Conscience* (Durham, N.C.: Duke University Press, 1961).

2. Thomas Aquinas, *Summa Theologica* II/II, Quest. XL, Art. 1.

3. Alfred Vanderpol, *La Doctrine scholastique du droit de guerre* (Paris: A. Pedone, 1919), 250ff.

4. The 1928 Pact of Paris, the "agreement to outlaw war," outlawed only first resort to force to settle international disputes; it did not abridge the right of use of force in self-defense. Similarly, the United Nations Charter, in articles 2 and 51, restricts the first use of force while continuing to reserve the right of second—defensive—use. For discussion see Henri Meyrowitz, *Le Principe de l'égalité des belligérents devant le droit de la guerre* (Paris: A. Pedone, 1970); Morton A. Kaplan and Nicholas deB. Katzenbach, "Resort to Force:

116   Johnson

War and Neutrality," in Richard A. Falk and Saul H. Mendlovitz, eds., *The Strategy of World Order,* vol. 2, *International Law* (New York: World Law Fund, 1966); and Johnson, *Ideology, Reason, and the Limitation of War,* 266–70.

5. The 1982 conflict between the United Kingdom and Argentina over the Falklands/ Malvinas Islands is a case in point. Both parties to this conflict argued that they were defending their own rights. Yet Argentina also justified its seizure of the Falklands/Malvinas as recovery of territory wrongly taken by the British 150 years earlier, and Britain in turn justified its military response as action to retake lost territory that was its own. Prime Minister Thatcher and her representatives also made much of the need to punish military aggression, while an undertone rose from among Third World countries that Argentina's action had been right because it was punishment of British colonialism. Here we have all three of the classic just causes (defense, recovery of something wrongly taken, punishment of evil) enumerated by Thomas Aquinas. Yet international law explicitly legitimizes only defense, and whatever the moral force of the other arguments, the legal case had to be put in these terms.

6. National Conference of Catholic Bishops, *The Challenge of Peace: God's Promise and Our Response* (Washington, D.C.: United States Catholic Conference, 1983).

7. It is, of course, a major theme in antinuclear writing to argue for the inherent disproportionality of nuclear weapons, as in, for example, Jonathan Schell, *The Fate of the Earth* (New York: Alfred Knopf, 1982). A more moderate position, nonetheless resting heavily on the argument from the disproportionality of such weapons, is exemplified by *The Challenge of Peace.* See pars. 152–53, 180, 184, 189.

8. See, for example, Alan Geyer, *The Idea of Disarmament!* (Elgin, Ill.: Brethren Press, 1982), 191–93; and John Howard Yoder, *When War Is Unjust* (Minneapolis, Minn.: Augsburg Publishing House, 1984), 79–80.

9. O'Brien, *Just and Limited War,* explictly makes this point in chs. 3 and 8.

10. James F. Childress, *Moral Responsibility in Conflicts* (Baton Rouge: Louisiana State University Press, 1982), ch. 3.

11. Paul Ramsey comments on the need to recover "the memory of a distinction" between combatants and noncombatants; see his *The Just War* (New York: Charles Scribner's Sons, 1968), chs. 7, 17. On the linkage between the justification of strategic bombing in World War II and nuclear strategy after 1945, see Lawrence Freedman, *The Evolution of Nuclear Strategy* (New York: St. Martin's Press, 1981), ch. 1; cf. my *Can Modern War Be Just?* (New Haven, Conn.: Yale University Press, 1984), 129–38.

12. See Freedman, *Nuclear Strategy,* chs. 4, 15–16, and passim; and Michael Mandelbaum, *The Nuclear Question* (Cambridge: Cambridge University Press, 1979), chs. 3–4.

13. See notes 1 and 11.

14. See *The Challenge of Peace,* par. 81.

15. Ibid., pars. 188, 190.

16. Yoder, *When War Is Unjust,* 64–67.

17. See further my exploration of this implication of just-war tradition in *Can Modern War Be Just?,* chs. 3, 5.

18. See "Obstacles Force Narrower Focus on 'Star Wars,' " *New York Times* (October 19, 1986), 1.

19. See, for example, Zbigniew Brzezinski, Robert Jastrow, and Max M. Kampelman, "Defense in Space Is Not 'Star Wars,' " *New York Times Magazine* (January 27, 1985), 28–29, 46, 48, 51.

20. *New York Times* (March 7, 1985), 1, A24.

21. Ibid. (October 19, 1986), 1, 14.

22. For further development of this line of reasoning, see *Can Modern War Be Just?*, 112–21, 138–48.

23. Whether a given individual is a combatant depends on actions, not attitudes. In the eighteenth century, Emmerich de Vattel put the argument this way: "Women, children, the sick and aged, are in the number of enemies. . . . But these are members [of the enemy society] who make no resistance, and consequently give us no right to treat their persons ill, or use any violence against them, much less to take away their lives." Emmerich de Vattel, *The Law of Nations; or Principles of the Law of Nature*, book 3, section 145.

24. For a concise discussion of the requirements of the just-war *jus in bello* and its connection to the international law of war, see O'Brien, *Just and Limited War*, ch. 3.

25. Ramsey, *War and the Christian Conscience*, 148–49, 228–29, 232–33, 260–64, 320–23; cf. Michael Walzer, *Just and Unjust Wars* (New York: Basic Books, 1977), ch. 17, and O'Brien, *Just and Limited War*, 47–48, 128, 135, 137–39, 343–44.

26. Thomas Powers, "Nuclear Winter and Nuclear Strategy," *Atlantic Monthly* (November 1984), 55.

27. These figures are taken from Michael F. Altfield and Stephen J. Cimbala, "Targeting for Nuclear Winter: A Speculative Essay," *Parameters: Journal of the U.S. Army War College* 15, no. 3 (Autumn 1985): 10.

28. The phrase is the title of ch. 1 in Schell's *Fate of the Earth*.

29. Altfield and Cimbala, "Nuclear Winter," 10.

The Discussion in
West Germany

6 • Problems of Method and Moral Theory in the U.S. and German Catholic Pastoral Letters on Peace: A Comparative Explanation

JOHN LANGAN, S.J.

I

The meeting of the U.S. Catholic bishops in Chicago in May 1983 at which the final version of *The Challenge of Peace,* their pastoral letter on war and peace, was approved by an overwhelming majority was probably the high point of public interest in this document. One indication of the level of public interest was the fact that while there were 300 bishops at the meeting, over 600 journalists from around the world covered the final discussion of the document. The letter itself pronounced on the world's foremost political concern, nuclear weapons—a subject of formidable complexity and controversy—from the perspective of a rich and flexible theological tradition which was, however, alien to many of the millions who would rely on journalistic accounts.

Most of the journalists, many of the concerned policy makers, and the bulk of the public were most interested in what stand the bishops would take on the "bottom line" issues of "no first use" of nuclear weapons, the legitimacy of fighting an extended nuclear war, and the moral status of nuclear deterrence, since these were the issues that could lead to direct conflict with U.S. government policy and that might well trigger crises of conscience for Catholics and others serving in the U.S. armed forces or involved in the development and production of nuclear weapons. The bishops themselves had to be concerned primarily with the fidelity of their document to the word of God and the teaching of the church and with its adequacy to the demands of the situation confronting reflective decision makers and conscientious Christians. They were acting as leaders of a church with a universal moral teaching, with a strong sense of institutional memory and international responsibility, and with a very diverse flock ranging from Pentagon officials to pacifist members of the Catholic

Worker Movement. But other groups were also deeply interested in the deliberations in Chicago and in the remarkable process of consultation and debate that had shaped the document over the previous two years. Among these were Catholic hierarchies in other countries that had strong concerns over U.S. strategic policy.

The bishops of the Federal Republic of Germany had already prepared a weighty document of their own on this subject, and the French hierarchy was in the process of doing so. Eventually over twenty Catholic hierarchies, including those of such nonnuclear powers as Ireland, Hungary, and Japan, issued pronouncements on this subject.[1] The Vatican itself had shown its special interest in the document at a meeting with leaders of the U.S. hierarchy and the drafting committee in Rome in March 1983. Church leaders, theologians, and peace activists in other Christian traditions were also anxious to assess the final version of the document. They had already been concerned witnesses to the debate on nuclear policy in the Church of England in 1982–83.[2] Many church groups were planning statements of their own on these matters, which would be either complementary to or critical of the Catholic effort.

Scholars from a variety of disciplines were deeply interested as well in how the document would deal with an issue that had proved to be profoundly intractable in both theoretical and practical terms. Their interest was as much in the coherence and adequacy of the argument and in the conceptual categories and intellectual resources used in making the argument as it was in specific policy conclusions. Biblical scholars, moral theologians and philosophers, students of Soviet society and Soviet-American relations, strategic theorists and writers on deterrence, international lawyers and military historians, political theorists, and experts on peace movements all were anxious to see how the document would make use of experiences and insights and methods drawn from their various fields and whether it would say things that supported or contradicted their own conclusions. Indeed, the pastoral letter, along with the parallel German and French documents, has been the occasion for the production of a vast popular and scholarly literature.

Given the high level of public visibility that the pastoral letters achieved and the breadth of the interests that they touched, it was natural for scholars who had been involved in various ways in the process of preparing the German and U.S. letters to welcome an opportunity to come together for a more direct and concentrated dialogue. Media interpretations of the German and U.S. letters tended to present them in polar terms: right vs. left, anti-Soviet vs. anti-Reagan, traditional vs. innovative, acceptable to Rome vs. corrected by Rome, historically sophisticated vs. historically ignorant, doctrine oriented vs. policy oriented, closed vs. open. In this polarized interpretation, the German letter had the first position in each pair, and the U.S. letter had the second. Favorable or unfavorable judgments were either implied or explicitly asserted depending on which set of characteristics the reporter or critic preferred. This, it may safely be said, was a situation very likely to lead to mistrust between the two hierarchies and to misunderstanding among the general public, many of whom took the mistaken view that the U.S. bishops were on the verge of condemning nuclear deterrence and that the German bishops took a complaisant attitude to the dangers of nuclear war. At the same time, the two letters were clearly different in their processes of preparation, their methods of argument, their emphases, and their impact in the political debate within their respective countries. Some of the differences were obvious and fitted the journalistic polarization just mentioned. But some of them lay at much deeper levels, and were the kinds of matters that would repay scholarly scrutiny.

So it was not surprising that in late 1984 an inquiry came from representatives of the German bishops' conference to the U.S. Catholic Conference about the possibility of a dialogue between staff people and consultants and experts who had assisted in the internal discussions about the two letters. It was agreed that this dialogue would be more helpful if it was less formal than an official exchange between the two conferences. The Woodstock Theological Center was asked to serve as the coordinating organization on the U.S. side. The dialogue began with a meeting in Washington, D.C., in March 1985, which took as its starting point a series of questions prepared by the two sides.

The U.S. participants included Father Bryan Hehir, the principal adviser to the U.S. Catholic Conference in this area; Professor Bruce Russett of Yale University, a political scientist who had been deeply involved in the drafting process; Dr. Victor Alessi of the Arms Control and Disarmament Agency; Professor William O'Brien of Georgetown University, an expert on international law and just-war theory who had been both a witness before the drafting committee chaired by Cardinal Bernardin and a vocal critic of some aspects of the letter; Professor James Daugherty of St. Joseph's University in Philadelphia, a political scientist particularly concerned with new weapons technologies and international agencies; Father Charles Curran, a moral theologian who had testified before the Bernardin committee and who was then professor at the Catholic University of America; Mr. Edward Dougherty, a retired foreign service officer and adviser on political-military affairs for the U.S. Catholic Conference; Father Thomas Gannon, S.J., who was then the director of the Woodstock Theological Center; and myself, who became acting director of Woodstock before the second meeting.

The German group was led by Father Franz Böckle, who was professor of moral theology in the Catholic faculty at the University of Bonn and also at the time rector of the university and who had been a major drafter of the German bishops' letter. He was accompanied by Dr. Heinz-Theo Risse of the staff of the German bishops' conference and Father Hans Langendörfer, S.J., who was at that time assistant to Professor Böckle in Bonn and who is now on the staff of the federal chancellor. The German delegation also included a working group from the Hessian Institute for Peace Research in Frankfurt: Dr. Gerd Krell, Hans-Joachim Schmidt, and Thomas Risse-Kuppen, as well as Professor Ernst-Otto Czempiel, a political scientist at the University of Frankfurt, and Professor Bernard Fraling, a moral theologian from the University of Würzburg.

The two groups were quickly able to establish an excellent working rapport and to come to a shared understanding of many of the distinctive features of the two letters and the different ways in which they were interpreted and used in their respective religious and political contexts. For instance, within the U.S. bishops' conference there is a group of fifty to sixty bishops who have declared their commitment to Pax Christi and who occupy positions ranging from nuclear pacifism to a comprehensive theological pacifism. This segment of opinion within the conference was represented on the Bernardin committee by Bishop Thomas Gumbleton, who served for many years as an auxiliary bishop in Detroit but who has considerable influence in articulating a more radical approach to social justice issues. The absence of any comparable group within the German bishops' conference meant that there was in the German letter much less concern to find formulations that would be minimally acceptable to pacifist opinion as a sign of progress toward the ultimate renunciation of violence.

The members of the German conference, many of whom have previously served as university professors of theology, naturally gravitate to a more academic mode of presentation and are less concerned with communicating their conclusions in forms that require the simplification of complex issues. This contrast, however, should not be drawn too sharply, for both conferences had to ensure that their documents were adequate to the complexities of a difficult subject and were intelligible to educated nontheologians who were willing to make a serious effort to understand. Cultural differences between German and U.S. society—the special weight attached to expert opinion and the prestige of the professoriat in Germany, the special value accorded to open public discussion and to freedom of conscience and the continued anxieties about religious intrusions into politics in the United States—produced important differences between the two letters, in both procedure and context.

The influence of political and strategic differences can also be discerned in the way the German and U.S. debates crisscrossed. The Federal Republic, along with other allies of the United States in Europe, had to work through the high levels of political controversy provoked by the decision to deploy cruise missiles and Pershing II ballistic missiles as a response to the Soviet deployment of intermediate nuclear weapons in Eastern Europe. These are the weapons whose removal on both sides has been agreed to in the INF Treaty signed by Reagan and Gorbachev in Washington in December 1987. The United States was more concerned about the continuing defense buildup begun in the Carter administration and accelerated in the Reagan administration and about what many perceived as a greater willingness of the United States to use force in the resolution of international disputes. Like other Europeans, the Germans and particularly their political elites have been especially concerned about maintaining the U.S. commitment to extended deterrence, whereas Americans have been most anxious about the possibility of escalation to an unlimited thermonuclear war, which would devastate the United States as well as Europe and much of the Soviet Union. There are and will remain important differences in the ways in which the risks and evils of war are customarily conceived in the two societies, differences which have tested the skill and imagination of leaders within the Western alliance, particularly since the time of General de Gaulle.

The reception of the two documents in both societies revealed an interesting set of affinities between the German letter and U.S. conservatives on the one hand, and between the U.S. letter and West German Social Democrats on the other. German Social Democrats, despite the fact that the alliance decision to deploy the intermediate-range missiles with nuclear warheads was a policy originally promoted by Helmut Schmidt, the last Social Democratic chancellor, welcomed the insistence in the U.S. letter on the moral urgency of nuclear disarmament and on the dangers of any resort to nuclear weapons. U.S. conservatives applauded the strong emphasis of the German letter on the wider ideological issues, the more critical view of Marxism and of the Soviet Union, and what they regarded as its more robust justification of deterrence. It is also safe to say that leaders of the U.S. Catholic hierarchy were anxious about the possibility that their document would be regarded as a partisan political statement. This contrasts with the common expectation in the Federal Republic that there will be a general congruence between the social teachings of the Catholic bishops and the political values of the Christian Democrat–Christian Social coalition, which has been the dominant power in West German politics over the last forty years.

These differences, however, while they emerged clearly in the course of our conversations and are important for the understanding of the place of the two documents in the church life and the political life of their respective societies, were not the primary focus of our attention, which in the Washington meeting turned particularly to questions of method and moral theory. Answering such questions forced us into a careful reexamination of the text of the letters and of the precise ways in which arguments were made. It also required us to situate the letters within the context of contemporary Catholic moral theology and to ponder the paradox of how the U.S. letter, with its reliance on just-war theory and its avoidance of proportionalism in moral reasoning, led to a document that was more radical in its policy implications than the German letter.

The following section of this essay is my effort to work some of the major points that emerged in the course of our Washington dialogue into a more systematic statement of the differences between the two letters. An earlier form of this material served as the starting point for a second dialogue, with a slightly different list of participants, that we had in Bonn in September 1986 and that produced a series of papers that are to be published in the future. Readers should understand that I rely heavily on the insights of my partners in the dialogue but that the responsibility for the final formulation and for the interpretative framework is mine. The interpretative framework is taken from contemporary moral philosophy, though it is also commonly used in much of moral theology and Christian ethics.

II

In what follows, I will consider the different criteria and frameworks proposed for the moral assessment of nuclear deterrence and then some more specific questions about the two different patterns of argument and assessment found in the two letters.

It is characteristic of the German letter that it insists on the necessity of situating its assessment of security policy within the framework of peace policy. Security policy includes both political-legal and military elements. The German bishops state: "The aim of the military contribution towards the maintenance of peace under present conditions must not lie in the waging of war but in the preventing of war—and indeed of any warfare at all."[3] More specifically, they propose two standpoints for the ethical assessment of nuclear deterrence: "The first and decisive standpoint is the *goal* of this strategy, i.e., the prevention of war." The goal is presented as the only possible justification for the "enormous risks invariably attendant upon a nuclear arms build-up." The second standpoint "refers to the means, i.e., the envisaged conventional and nuclear weapons as well as the appropriate operational planning." The German bishops insist on the indispensability of assessing nuclear strategies and nuclear armaments in terms of the political objective. They then offer three specific criteria: (1) "existing or planned means must never render war more feasible or more probable," (2) "only such military means and so many military means may be deployed as are necessary for the purpose of the deterrent aimed at preventing war," and (3) "all military means must be compatible with effective mutual arms limitation, arms reduction, and disarmament." The German bishops admit that "the observance of these criteria does not furnish any absolute guarantee that deterrence reliably prevents war." They briefly consider the issue of what is to be done if deterrence fails. They call for political efforts to prevent hostilities and for the maintenance of communication between the two sides, and they denounce "automatism which emanates from the available weapons systems and proceeds to the decision makers." They repeat the Second Vatican Council's condemnation of the use of weapons of mass destruction against population centers and hold that "a war of destruction is never a solution and never permissible." They conclude that "mankind is now in an impasse," which requires "greater efforts toward a political maintenance of peace and continuous disarmament." They regard the toleration of deterrence so long as it prevents war as an instance of "choosing from among various evils the one which, as far as it is humanly possible to tell, appears the smallest," and they describe their statement of principles as "guided . . . by the precept of rationality."

Four general points need to be made about the German bishops' position on deterrence. First, it is a teleological position. Justification is provided by the end or the objective. Hence, the estimation of likely consequences and the reading of those factors in the context which can alter the consequences are extremely important in the argument and in practice. Among these contextual factors, the programs and procedures of the political order (both national and international) will have a central importance.

Second, it is not a utilitarian position if utilitarianism is understood as defining morally right action in terms of its ability to maximize a unique nonmoral good or even a set of nonmoral goods.[4] The objective is itself conceived in terms that include both the major moral values of the political order (freedom, human rights) and the major nonmoral harms (to life, property, the environment). The procedure that the German bishops employ does not involve justifying morally questionable means by appeals to a nonmoral end.

Third, the position taken in the German letter is proportionalist. Its willingness to allow the choice of a lesser evil presupposes some general ability to bring goods and evils under a general standard (not necessarily a standard capable of mathematical precision but rather one that is already present in our intelligent conduct of practical affairs). The concern, here as in proportionalism generally, is primarily with the outcomes to be produced or avoided rather than with the character of the actions by which these outcomes are brought about, though this concern is not excluded or dismissed.

Fourth, the order of the argument is to proceed from the teleological assessment of deterrence to the consideration, or perhaps better the non-consideration, of the problem of the moral assessment of the use of nuclear weapons. The German bishops do not proceed from the assessment of possible or proposed uses of nuclear weapons to the assessment of the threats to use them that are present in the system of deterrence. Accordingly, the *jus in bello* criteria of proportionality and discrimination do not play a fundamental part in their argument.

If we compare the U.S. bishops' letter with the German letter on these points, we arrive at the following conclusions. First, the U.S. letter also offers a teleological assessment of deterrence, though this matter is handled in an ambiguous fashion. The key passage here is paragraph 175:

> The moral duty today is to prevent nuclear war from ever occurring and to protect and preserve those key values of justice, freedom, and independence which are necessary for personal dignity and national integrity. In reference to these issues, Pope John Paul II judges that deterrence may still be judged morally acceptable, certainly, not as an end in itself but as a step on the way toward a progressive disarmament.[5]

Here I suggest that, despite the deontological language ("moral duty"), there is a double pattern of teleological justification at work. The point being made by the use of deontological language is that the ends are morally imperative, not merely optional or worthy but urgently necessary. The claim made in this paragraph, then, is that these two logically distinct and potentially separable ends provide moral justification for the risky and objectionable policy of deterrence and for the weapons systems and strategies that compose it. But there is also present in the text a more forward-looking argument which offers justification for deterrence as a temporary condition, a step on the way to disarmament. This is a different goal, one specified in negative terms but logically compatible with the double goal that is to be attained in the present and in the immediate future. There is, however, an important element of paradox here, for the further goal (disarmament) requires the renunciation of the means to the immediate double goal.

On the second point, we can see that the double goal includes both moral and nonmoral elements and that the U.S. bishops' position is not a pure utilitarianism. Whether it is a form of proportionalism is less clear. If one holds that the bishops should have judged deterrence to be a morally objectionable or morally flawed means to protect national values and to prevent war and that they are implicitly allowing the worth of the double end to justify a suspect means (not merely a means with some negative features or costs but simply a morally wrong means), then one has to hold that their argument is proportionalist. Certainly, they express the desire to get beyond reliance on this means, again borrowing words from John Paul II to this effect: "The logic of nuclear deterrence cannot be considered a final goal or an appropriate and secure means for safeguarding international peace." Settling this issue would, I think, require deciding whether the U.S. bishops' position is theoretically unified and coherent. We should also bear in mind that paragraph 106, which does not explicitly mention deterrence but speaks instead of "the arms race" (which could perhaps be restricted to the acquisition of new weapons but could also be applied to a more stable situation of mutual deterrence), envisions the possibility of a negative judgment about means "not evil in themselves" but disproportionate because of "attendant evils." The preceding paragraph speaks of means "evil in themselves," which no end can justify, and offers as examples "the executing of hostages or the targeting of non-combatants."

The fourth point, however, is one on which there is clear divergence between the German and U.S. approaches to the moral assessment of deterrence. For as is well known, the U.S. debate, shaped largely but not exclusively by the drafts of the bishops' letter, treated the assessment of nuclear deterrence as logically dependent on the assessment of the use of nuclear weapons. In the assessment of use, the bishops relied on the norms of the just-war doctrine (which are restated in contemporary terms in paragraphs 80–110). Particularly important are the *jus in bello* principles of proportionality and discrimination. The U.S. letter acknowledges that there is room for debate about the interpretation and application of both of these principles. The question then arises as to the status and character of these norms of just-war doctrine. Clearly, applying the norm of proportionality requires us to assess and compare advantages and disadvantages resulting from a policy or a particular course of action. Should the principle of discrimination be taken as enunciating an absolute prohibition of certain kinds of actions and therefore of policies of which they would form a constitutive part? Or should it be interpreted as an element in a proportionalist theory of moral reasoning in general or of just-war doctrine in particular so that it will function as an element for regulating violence in a way that will minimize harm to persons?

It seems clear to me that the U.S. bishops espouse the first possibility and that they do not allow proportionally grounded exceptions to the principle of discrimination. Whether they are correct in this is, of course, a matter for theoretical argument; but it seems to me that their view is in the mainstream of historical Catholic thinking about moral rules. They are effectively treating the principle of discrimination as an exceptionless moral rule, though they are prepared to allow some indeterminacy in the application of this norm and to accept some indirect killing of civilians (to be limited by the principle of proportionality, which is present in applications of the principle of double effect).

It seems, however, that paragraph 149 of the U.S. letter could be read as pointing to the possibility of interpreting the principle of discrimination on proportionalist lines. In this interpretation, they would be reaffirming and strengthening the principle of discrimination against the erosion which it has suffered in recent times on the slippery slope of modern technological forms of warfare.

We should also note that the U.S. bishops not only speak of the killing of civilians as a means wrong in itself but also explicitly mention "the targeting of non-combatants." This brings up the complex connections between targeting policy on the one hand and threat and intention on the other. But it would be a plausible reading of this passage to see it as condemning explicit and implicit threats to kill noncombatants directly and thus as rejecting a certain range of ways of implementing deterrence, precisely for the reason that it is wrong to threaten to do what is wrong to do. This principle for assessing the morality of threats has been challenged by various philosophers and is explicitly rejected in the French bishops' letter.[6]

Just what specific evaluations of the use of nuclear weapons follow from the two *jus in bello* principles of proportionality and discrimination? The U.S. bishops, following on this point the teaching of the Second Vatican Council (which, as already seen, is also found in the German letter), condemned the destruction of cities and population centers, even in retaliation. This is a fairly straightforward application of the principle of discrimination. The bishops also rejected the first use of nuclear weapons. This is a judgment which relies decisively on the danger of escalation to a level which would violate the principle of proportionality. It is a judgment which the bishops explicitly place in the set of "prudential judgments . . . based on specific circumstances which can change or . . . be interpreted differently by people of good will" (par. 10). The bishops make a number of statements which converge in support of their negative judgment about the first use of nuclear weapons and which, taken together, suggest that the "fragile barrier—political, psychological, and moral—which has been constructed since 1945" against the use of nuclear weapons (par. 153) should be treated as an absolute prohibition. But their argument never achieves the status of strict demonstration (in which one who accepts the premises must accept the conclusion). In line with their negative judgment on first use, they also adopt a very skeptical view of the possibility of conducting a limited nuclear war. They also base this view on the *jus ad bellum* requirement that there be "a reasonable hope of success in bringing about justice and peace" (par. 159). They do not consider those scenarios in which nonuse either as a declaratory policy or as an actual course of events has a negative effect on the prospects for bringing about justice and peace, except for their recognition of the need to find alternative modes of defense to prevent a conventional attack by the Soviet Union in Europe (par. 155).

The negative positions that the U.S. bishops offer on both the first use of nuclear weapons and the prospects for fighting a limited nuclear war rely on a reasonable (though not demonstrative) judgment that excessive harm would result. This sort of judgment requires some sort of prudential calculus and a commensuration of different kinds of harms and benefits. The argument is not made (though it could be) that the evil of such use of nuclear weapons consists in its leading to direct attacks on population centers as a result of the political pressures that leaders would be under, especially if the question arose of retaliating against enemy attacks on population centers. This sort of judgment, however, does not require that those who make it treat all the norms of just-war theory on proportionalist lines, but it does seem to be incompatible with some of the more sweeping attacks on proportionalism as a method of moral reasoning.[7] It also allows for the possibility of a changed context in which different judgments, both about the likelihood of escalation and about the moral justifiability of the use of nuclear weapons, might be reached. Such a changed context is necessarily presupposed when we shift from considering the use of nuclear weapons by the superpowers against each other to other possible situations involving nuclear or near-nuclear powers, such as Israel, though this is not a topic that either letter treats explicitly.

The judgments which the U.S. bishops' letter offers about possible uses of nuclear weapons are not normative merely for courses of action that might be proposed and carried out in the event of hostilities between the superpowers or between NATO and the Warsaw Pact. They present a normative set of restrictions for the way in which a nuclear deterrent is to be structured. Taken together with the principle that it is wrong to threaten or to intend what it is wrong to do, they create a serious challenge to deterrence in general. As the bishops point out, "Still other observers, many of them Catholic moralists, have stressed that deterrence may not morally include the intention of deliberately attacking civilian populations or noncombatants" (par. 169).

The U.S. bishops go on to offer a general teleological justification for nuclear deterrence that relies on the authority of John Paul II and focuses on the double goal of preventing nuclear war and preserving the key moral-political values of "justice, freedom, and independence" (pars. 171–76). But this general, though qualified, endorsement of deterrence does not entail an acceptance of all forms of deterrence or of the legitimacy of the means involved in any particular form of deterrence. The U.S. bishops put the matter thus: "Although we acknowledge the need for [a] deterrent, not all forms of deterrence are morally acceptable. There are moral limits to deterrence policy as well as to policy regarding use. Specifically it is not morally acceptable to intend to kill the innocent as part of a strategy of deterring nuclear war" (par. 178).

The argument of the U.S. bishops indicates that they regard the prohibition against threats and intentions to attack innocent civilians as an exceptionless norm in the same way as they regard the prohibition against actually killing innocent civilians. It is worth pointing out that this equivalence holds only if the bridge principle—if doing X is morally wrong, then threatening to do X is morally wrong—is itself exceptionless. It is possible that the bridge principle linking use and threat holds true in general, but that it admits of some exceptions (of which deterrence in the defense of a just society might be one). One might argue that the institutional character of deterrence policy produces a gap between threat and action which makes application of the principle inappropriate.[8] Or one might argue that the burden of proof rests on those who would treat the principle as exceptionless, saying in effect that the principle as it is commonly presented is simply a useful rule of thumb. In any event, the point would remain that unless it is right to regard the bridge principle as exceptionless, the condemnation of deterrence on the ground that it involves immoral threats does not follow as a matter of strict logic.

Also, care should be taken to keep the following formulations distinct: (1) It is morally wrong to threaten to do what is morally wrong. (2) It is morally wrong to threaten to do X, which is in fact morally wrong. The second formulation would allow for a separate evaluation of the threat and its implementation. The case for separate evaluation rests on the separability of the two actions in the real order and on the agent's negative attitude to actual implementation, which is significantly different from the standard situation in voluntary action, in which there is a direct unilinear movement from intention to implementation. Making this point is not to deny that there is an element of paradox in any conclusion of this general form: (3) It is morally right to threaten to do X, which is in fact morally wrong.

These refinements aside, the general tendency of the U.S. position is clear: it is to restrict the range of threats in any deterrence policy to those actions which it would be moral to carry out as this is determined by the *jus in bello* norms of just-war theory. Considerations of whether such a restricted range of threats would damage the ability of deterrence policy to achieve its moral-political goals of preventing war and preserving the key values of justice, freedom, and independence are subordinated to the moral requirements of just-war theory. This position of the U.S. bishops accords with a standard pattern of situations of moral crisis in deontological approaches to moral thinking: obedience to an exceptionless moral norm conflicts with the attainment of a worthy goal and may in fact require the sacrifice of that goal.

This pattern conforms to the widespread expectation in common, pre-theoretical conceptions of morality that doing the right thing can have serious costs and may indeed require heavy sacrifices. It is supported by the contrast that many thinkers in the modern period have drawn between self-interest and morality. It is familiar, and it also provides a basis for interpreting what saints and heroes do in laying down their lives in fidelity to moral principle or moral values. While this pattern is familiar and welcome in understanding the moral crises of individuals, it is more problematic in interpreting the moral crises of entire societies or of humanity in general. Both utilitarians and state moralists (of whom Michael Walzer is the most influential recent U.S. example) would regard it as mistaken and perhaps even as absurd.

The subordination of what is ordinarily taken to be the political form of the common good to the norms of just-war theory is a move which the U.S. bishops are willing to make and which some prominent Catholic moralists (Anscombe, Grisez, and Finnis) are willing to endorse explicitly. But for Walzer and for many utilitarians, it is unacceptable and perhaps even unintelligible. His unwillingness to make this move, combined with his view that deterrence policy is incompatible with the just-war norms, leads Walzer to offer his proposal for legitimating deterrence as a kind of supreme emergency. We should also observe that a utilitarian approach to contemporary security problems may take the form of subordinating the key values of common political life in a system of nation-states to ensure the continued survival of humanity (possibly through the reconstruction of the entire political order, as proposed, for instance, by Jonathan Schell[9], or possibly through accommodation on the best terms attainable from our adversaries, if the emphasis is on an immediate resolution of the problem and if we make the not unreasonable supposition that they are unwilling to give up their own nuclear forces).

The U.S. bishops, however, do not wish to be backed into a corner on this matter. Their recommendation, their hope, is to find a form of deterrence policy that does not violate the norms of discrimination and proportionality, is limited to sufficiency, and is conducive to progressive disarmament (par. 188). This position, as the bishops recognize, commits them to a stance of critical revisionism with regard to the actual form of U.S. deterrence policy and will require a "substantial intellectual, political, and moral effort" (par. 196).

The first requirement is that the threatened actions in a deterrence policy not violate the principle of discrimination and, thus, that nuclear weapons not be targeted at "civilian centers" (par. 178). This requirement is partially met by U.S. declaratory policy which refrains from targeting "the Soviet civilian population as such" and which does not propose "to use nuclear weapons deliberately for the purpose of destroying population centers" (par. 179). But the U.S. bishops also insist that this requirement is insufficient. They are concerned about the prospect of "indirect, (i.e., unintended) but massive civilian casualties" which would result from attacks on military and industrial targets which are, as they observe, "thoroughly interspersed with civilian living and working areas" (par. 180). These possibilities are to be assessed, they say, by "a different moral criterion: the principle of proportionality" (par. 180).

They acknowledge that judgments of proportionality are "always open to different evaluations," but they affirm that "there are actions which can be decisively judged to be disproportionate" (par. 181). They do not provide examples to illustrate this interesting and plausible claim, and so it is unclear whether they have in mind primarily a specific action, such as exploding an atomic bomb over a weapons factory in Moscow, or a series of actions. But what does seem to be clear is that the disproportionality, the excess of harm over benefit in relation to a specific goal in a given context, applies to the action or actions of using the weapons rather than to the making of threats, whether this be done by deployment and targeting or by explicit statements made to the adversary. It is clear that the real-life consequences of those actions can be and are significantly different from the consequences of making the threats. But the U.S. approach, which requires that we base assessment of threat on assessment of actual use, forbids us to consider this difference. It rules out a deterrence strategy which would, in the event of failure, produce disproportionate consequences.

This sort of judgment is, as the bishops would probably acknowledge, easier to make in retrospect. But such a judgment is not helpful as a guide to the formation of policy in the present. So the bishops are driven to bring into their assessments a probabilistic mode of reasoning. The concern of policy makers and of those who would offer them moral counsel must be not merely with the magnitude and the character of consequences but also with the likelihood of their occurrence. This consideration leads the U.S. bishops to take a negative view of more accurate weapons, which in their view would increase "the likelihood of escalation at a level where many, even 'discriminating' weapons would cumulatively kill very large numbers of civilians" (par. 183). They take a similarly negative view of "counterforce targeting" both because it is "often joined" with statements of declaratory policy that imply that a nuclear war can be fought within "precise rational and moral limits" and because of the threat that such a targeting policy presents to the forces of the other side, "making deterrence unstable in a crisis and war more likely" (par. 184). Here we find the bishops appealing to the likely consequences both of actual use (par. 183) and of threat and targeting policy (par. 184).

Now what is clearly fundamental in the bishops' argument here is not an individual judgment about the disproportionality of the use of nuclear weapons in a given context or even a series of such judgments but rather the negative judgment about the consequences of crossing the firebreak which led to their rejection of the first use of nuclear weapons. For the immediate consequences of using more discriminate nuclear weapons against military targets not only would conform to the principle of discrimination but also would be more in accordance with the principle of proportionality, since greater precision in targeting and restriction to military targets will reduce collateral damage.

The real concern of the U.S. bishops has to be about the consequences of the process of escalation once begun. This concern, while eminently reasonable and appropriate, brings with it a significantly different conception of proportionality than one would use in weighing the harms and benefits produced by a given action. It relies on a constant feature of the nuclear situation, namely the possibility of escalating to catastrophic levels at which the harms that would be produced would clearly outweigh any benefits that might reasonably be expected. At the same time, the connection between the various policies and actions both on the level of threat and on the level of use and the set of catastrophic consequences remains contingent and variable. This point is particularly important in assessing the intentions present in a deterrence policy, since most of these consequences will not be intended in the strict sense. It also involves a series of actions for which neither side in the conflict bears exclusive responsibility.

There are important differences between the consequences of an action considered in its immediate context (e.g., the removal of an ectopic pregnancy) where there is no *novus actus interveniens* and the consequences, broadly and even loosely conceived, of an action which is part of a complex interactive process.[10] The constant presence of catastrophic outcomes as possible results of various forms of deterrence policy is clearly a factor that should produce in all parties an attitude of concern and caution. Just how closely these possible negative outcomes can be tied to violations of the principle of proportionality is a matter on which I must profess both uncertainty and skepticism. At the least, I would maintain that the U.S. bishops' argument here needs fuller and more careful statement.

There is also need for reflection on the possibility that significant changes in the technology of command, control, communications, and intelligence might simultaneously increase the possibility of limited and discriminate nuclear exchanges while reducing the likelihood of catastrophic nuclear exchanges. This would challenge the U.S. bishops' reliance on the likelihood of escalation in their contention that shifting to a counterforce doctrine would be incompatible with the principle of proportionality.

In summary, then, it seems that the German letter leaves theorists with the freedom to construct arguments for forms of nuclear deterrence in which the importance of the goals to be attained or preserved provides justification for relying on means that are at variance with traditional moral rules. But it leaves unresolved the problem presented by the intentional linkage between negatively evaluated actions (morally wrong acts that violate just-war norms) and the legitimated threats to do such actions which are found in a strategy of deterrence. The U.S. letter, on the other hand, provides an extremely restricted basis for the justification of deterrence. The more specific norms of the U.S. letter, moreover, suffer from incomplete and inconsistent argumentation.

Notes

1. For an overview of these letters, see Mark Heirman, "Bishops' Conferences on War and Peace in 1983," *Cross Currents* 33 (1983): 275–87.

2. The debate in the general synod of the Church of England was about whether to accept the recommendations in *The Church and the Bomb,* the report of a working group headed by the Right Reverend John Austin Baker, Bishop of Salisbury. These recommendations included unilateral nuclear disarmament by the United Kingdom and were not accepted.

3. All references to the text of the German letter *Gerechtigkeit schafft Frieden* are to the English translation, *Out of Justice, Peace,* prepared by Irish Messenger Publications and edited by James V. Schall, S.J. (San Francisco: Ignatius Press, 1984).

4. See, for instance, the definition of utilitarianism given in the influential text of William Frankena, *Ethics,* 2d ed. (Englewood Cliffs, N.J.: Prentice-Hall, 1973), 34.

5. All references to the U.S. pastoral letter are to *The Challenge of Peace* (Washington, D.C.: United States Catholic Conference, 1983).

6. See *Gagner la paix,* translated as *Winning the Peace,* ed. James V. Schall, trans. Michael Wrenn (San Francisco: Ignatius Press, 1984), pars. 26–30.

7. As, for instance, in the recent work of John Finnis, Joseph M. Boyle, Jr., and Germain Grisez, *Nuclear Deterrence, Morality, and Realism* (Oxford: Clarendon Press, 1987).

8. This position has been argued in various places with different nuances by Michael Novak.

9. Jonathan Schell, *The Fate of the Earth* (New York: Alfred Knopf, 1982), 181–231.

10. Alan Donagan, *The Theory of Morality* (Chicago: University of Chicago Press, 1977), 43–52.

7 • Nuclear Weapons and Peace: Political Challenge and Theological Controversy in West German Protestantism

TRUTZ RENDTORFF

The Debate Within the Churches

A report on the discussion in the Federal Republic of Germany between theological ethicists and churches on the one hand and strategists and politicians on the other has to take into account at least three different points: (1) the general political context of the debate, (2) the theological context of the debate, and (3) the specific situation of Christians in Germany living in a nation divided between East and West. As to the general political context, the debate on nuclear weapons, nuclear deterrence, and the nuclear dilemma has taken place in two phases. In the late fifties the first great debate among Protestants in Germany was provoked by the question of rearmament under Chancellor Konrad Adenauer. The central issue then was whether the newly built-up army of the Federal Republic should have nuclear weapons.[1] The controversial issue of rearmament developed principally into a debate on the A-bomb as a morally legitimate means of defense. Nuclear strategy, at that time, was not well developed, and the churches, like other institutions, were still influenced by World War II. Increasing East-West tension tended toward a new military conflict. The argument on the nuclear issue was at the same time an argument on the dangers of Communist dominance in Germany. The fear of Communism represented the experience of the lost war. After 1945 the Soviet Union appeared on the European scene as one new superpower, the United States having become the other. Thus, in addition to controversies on rearmament, the attitude towards the liberal West over against the socialist East permeated all questions under debate. But the public debate became especially heated because of the German issue: What would be the consequences of reunification? Which decision would help the prospect of reunification? Which decision would support the division? The search for peace took place within the dilemma of "freedom" or "unity" for the Germans. One has to keep in mind these different factors in order to understand that the debate on the nuclear problem always implied much more than ethical judgment concerning military force. It was and still is a broad and far-reaching political issue including the whole range of problems arising from the twelve years of Nazi rule. In this perspective, a specific German problem strongly shapes the debate on nuclear armament. Already in this first phase it had become clear that ethical problems of nuclear armament could not be isolated from their political context.

When, in the second phase in the early eighties, the INF issue caused a new and very agitated public debate, the political discussion focused again on the position of the Federal Republic between East and West. As in the first phase, *peace* appeared to be the catchword for an orientation toward the East, implying that the root causes for a possible war were in the deployment of INF by the U.S. forces (although in the framework of NATO), whereas the political support for the INF decision was directly linked to a close relationship to the West and stressed the freedom of liberal democracies. And again political motives proved stronger than ethical judgments concerning the irresponsibility of nuclear warfare. The pressure of Soviet propaganda against the deployment of the new generation of weapons influenced a strong minority of voters, but the majority and the leading political forces viewed the anti-INF criticism from the East as a move to separate the Federal Republic from its allies and to end U.S. presence on German soil.

It is obvious that the political context of the nuclear debate is not symmetrical with the ethical questions nuclear weapons pose. In both phases the churches had great difficulty in deciding which issue should be given priority. The experience with the Third Reich had taught the Protestant churches that they should keep a clear distance from direct political involvement, that their ecclesiastical independence should forbid them either to vote solely for one party and against the other or to make their commitment politically too outspoken. But they could not avoid the fact that any position on the armament question implied, even if not intentionally so, a political decision within the East-West tension.

The debate in the late fifties found its most prominent expression in the discussion of the General Synod of the Evangelical Church in Germany, which at that time was the synod of all Protestant churches in both parts of the country. The synod did not reach consensus but had to state that there was a deep split among Protestants. The only way out was to confess that "we stay together" under the "gospel" in spite of deep differences in political ethics. Already it had become clear that a small but theologically powerful group of theologians and laypersons had decided that the question of rearmament in general and the nuclear issue in particular was leading toward a new *status confessionis*. They approached all questions believing that the Confessing Church, which had been formed as a defense against the Nazis, had to be continued in the postwar era. To them, the problem of the A-bomb was not only a challenge to political decisions but much more a question of the identity of the church. The majority, however, did not follow this theological judgment, preferring to look at these problems as worldly affairs to be judged according to criteria of human reasoning.

Politics in general and the military issue in particular initiated within the churches a debate on the role of the church. The different positions implied far-reaching, fundamental theological controversies. In this context one can identify the ambivalent role of Karl Barth and his theological influence. On the one hand, Barth was seen as the prominent figure who had taught the church to keep away from political involvement and to stick to the preaching of the word of God. On the other hand, he was the same man who already had taken a definite position on several political questions and who now voted against rearmament in Germany (but not against a Swiss army!). The focus of the debate within the churches and among theologians differed considerably from the general political and ethical debate. It has been over and over again a controversy about the consequences one had to draw from the church struggle and about the differences in the understanding of the Confessing Church.

Since the General Synod of the Evangelical Church in Germany did not come to a consensus, a small group of theologians and laypersons outside the synod issued a document known as the Heidelberg Theses of 1959.[2] In this statement the central idea of complementarity paved the way for a compromise within the churches. In an analogy to physics (and by quoting a concept of Niels Bohr) the statement formulated a complementarity of positions that seem to be antagonistic. In the same way that a physicist may identify light either as waves or as small particles, one can have different perspectives on the same issue, neither view necessarily excluding the other. They are both possible, each view representing parts of the whole truth. In that sense they are complementary.

This concept of complementarity was applied to the controversy within the church and among Christians: both attitudes—that condemning nuclear weapons and that tolerating them—are possible, and therefore Christians may be against participation in nuclear politics as well as for it. They are bound to each other.

The theological impact of complementarity is due to an eschatological perspective: under the conditions of a sinful world, which is "not yet" redeemed, it may "yet" be possible or even necessary for Christians to participate in military activities. At the same time, those who object to participation "already" give witness of the coming world. The complementarity of decisions exemplifies the eschatological tension.

This complementarity was taken up on all sides. For the churches it had a great pacifying function. Nevertheless, they reached no clear consensus regarding the period in which it "yet" should be possible for Christians to be part of military affairs and when this period would be over. On the one hand, this period was identified with the history of a sinful world until the Second Coming of Christ. On the other, it was perceived as a transition in which the abolition of nuclear weapons (and military force in general) had to be achieved—the sooner the better. So there remained a latent conflict that broke out anew in the early eighties.

At the beginning of the INF debate, the Council of the Evangelical Church in Germany decided to state publicly the position of the Protestant Church. They asked their Commission for Public Responsibility to prepare a memorandum on the peace issue. This commission includes politicians, academics, theologians, and church leaders representing different parties and various political and theological strands within West German Protestantism. At that time, the churches in the German Democratic Republic had already separated from the Evangelical Church in Germany, setting up their own ecclesiastical institutions.

The commission drafted a memorandum entitled "The Preservation, Promotion and Renewal of Peace," which was published in October 1981 with the full approval of the church government. The memorandum took a very clear line. It took its start from an analysis of the situation of world politics and aimed at the political task of peacemaking as the primary ethical issue. It warned against a purely military perspective and expressed the conviction that the debate within the church and in public was badly advised if it estimated military strategies and advanced military technology to be the main dangers. The memorandum called for a new political perspective to regain that dimension of the present conflict; it argued against the ethical debate's dominating focus on military force. The ethical question had to be reformulated. Public discussion within the church and beyond underrated the political task of preserving, promoting, and renewing peace under conditions of antagonism and over-rated the role of weaponry. The document further challenged the churches to influence the political ethos and to develop concepts of coop-eration that might have a better chance against the language of weapons. Within this context the memorandum indirectly reaffirmed the concept of complementarity.[3]

This document found wide reception among the churches and repre-sents the mainline position of the Protestant churches in West Germany today. It served as a platform with which to keep balance in the contro-versies resulting from the formation of the peace movement.

In 1983, the German Bishops Conference of the Roman Catholic Church in West Germany published a "Word" to its members under the title *Gerechtigkeit schafft Frieden (Out of Justice, Peace).*[4] This state-ment was influenced by the memorandum of the Evangelical Church and was, in its latest stages, a response to the 1983 pastoral letter of the U.S. bishops. The position taken by the German bishops differed from that of the U.S. bishops insofar as it concentrated on the ethical concept of jus-tice and discussed the political responsibility to establish an international order of peace. The statement took the same line the memorandum al-ready had taken. The primary problem is not one of nuclear weapons as such but is a problem of political order under conditions of antagonistic political systems. The political situation creates the tensions that are expressed in the nuclear debate. The Catholic and Protestant churches of West Germany therefore took similar positions in the general controversy, regardless of differences in theological traditions and ethical language. The debate in the Roman Catholic Church kept clearly away from a con-fessional argument and stuck to rational ones of political ethics, as the authors of the Protestant memorandum had tried to do. But the Protestant memorandum was less successful.

In this controversy a statement of the Reformed Convention (Re-formierter Bund), an association of congregations and individual Prot-estants of the Reformed Church, was issued in 1982.[5] This statement pro-claimed a *status confessionis* as the church's position against nuclear weapons. Under the title *Das Bekenntnis zu Jesus Christus und die Frie-*

densverantwortung der Kirche (The Confession to Jesus Christ and the Responsibility of the Church for Peace), this statement pronounced that for the church the nuclear question is not a political question but a question of faith and of confession, on the same level as the confession to Jesus Christ. Starting from the Christian confession of God's reconciliation with the world in the death and resurrection of Jesus Christ, the statement draws direct political and ethical consequences from dogmatic sentences, which lead to an uncompromising "no" to nuclear weapons together with all military force. In the judgment of the Reformed Church, nuclear pacifism has become a dividing line between true and false theology. In the INF debate, this statement gained broad public recognition and renewed the discussion of the late fifties. Various proposals were brought forward to associate the *status confessionis* with different strategic options for nuclear-free zones in Europe or for alternative defense concepts. But there was no consensus with regard to the theological presuppositions the Reformed Church made. The theological debate tended to function as a cover for political positions. Finally, the discussion made clear that the controversy centered on the problem of whether nuclear weapons were to be considered "political weapons" bound up in the concept of deterrence or whether they were to be negated on ethical and theological grounds, regardless of their political function.

The churches in the German Democratic Republic took a different route.[6] They engaged very strongly in the peace issue and came to the point where their position was very much in accordance with the politics of the East. They increasingly found government approval in teaching the renunciation of the spirit and logic of deterrence. In a number of resolutions by the General Synod of the Churches in East Germany this formula developed into a kind of confession: *The Renunciation of the Spirit and Logic of Deterrence.* The churches in the Democratic Republic were at first unaware that deterrence, particularly nuclear deterrence, was a strategic concept that had been developed by the West and that had never been formally adopted as official Soviet military doctrine. Therefore the renunciation of deterrence could be tolerated and even supported by the state authorities, since the refusal of the explicit concept of deterrence moved in the same direction as the official politics against the security concept of NATO. The churches therefore later added to their formula the word *practice*, so that the position is now entitled *The Renunciation of the Spirit, Logic and Practice of Deterrence.* Although it was obvious that the East

German churches, like the Russian Orthodox Church, stood in line with the political struggle of the East against the deployment of the INF weapons by NATO, their main point was to strengthen their position as churches within a socialist state. Until the United States and the Soviet Union reached an agreement on the removal of all INF weapons from Europe, there was a growing, although carefully hedged, disagreement among the Protestant churches in East as well as West Germany. The theological debate, at any rate, did not come to the point of direct confrontation. There had been some efforts to transform the renunciation formula into a direct confession in the sense of a *status confessionis*, using the term *renunciation* with the meaning it had had in the teaching of the baptism (renunciation of the devil). But this attempt did not become an official position of the church in East Germany.

The East German church also started the initiative for a worldwide peace council at the World Assembly of the World Council of Churches in Vancouver. This idea of a council marks the last stage in the church debate on peace and nuclear weapons. In 1985, at the Kirchentag in Düsseldorf, a proclamation was published asking the churches in the world to call a "Council of Peace." The idea's promoter, Carl Friedrich von Weizsäcker, was the author of the Heidelberg Theses of 1959. He confessed publicly that he had lost any confidence in politicians but felt encouraged by the peace movement that a conversion of consciousness among people might now be possible, providing an adequate way to promote a general change of peace politics. But when this idea emerged, it became clear that the peace issue had already lost its primary significance and that ecological problems and, even more, problems of economic justice in the Third World had come to the fore. The conciliar process which is now going on therefore combines all relevant issues of the world of today. The conferences which are arranged to prepare the way for an ecumenical convocation include a range of items, as expressed in its program "Justice, Peace and the Preservation of Creation." The nuclear question is no longer the central point of controversy but is one topic among others.

The periodic dramatization of the nuclear dilemma clearly shows that the churches and theologians have great difficulties in coming to grips with political and ethical problems that cannot be identified in terms of a sharp church/state, faith/world distinction but that rather result from the involvement of Christians in issues which cross the divides of such distinctions. Theologians and the churches find themselves in a situation in which they must determine how they can bring their special message into responsible dialogue with the responsibilities stemming from the task of worldly politics.

One enduring topic of major importance has been the teaching of just war. The next section will discuss how this teaching may be reformulated under the conditions and from the perspective of nuclear deterrence.

Ethical Problems of the Just-War Doctrine

Two problem areas in particular which prevent a simple readoption and continuation of the just-war doctrine in peace ethics today must be emphasized.

The Proportionality of Means and Ends in the Nuclear Age

The limiting nature of the just-war doctrine, as conceived in the notion *jus in bello*, was already a problem in World War I and much more so in World War II; indeed, it was shaken to its foundations. The waging of war with means and strategies of mass destruction is an inexorable feature of the political and ethical discussion of peace.

In World War II the distinction between combatants and noncombatants, important for the concept of *jus in bello*, was effectively undermined. Wars waged as wars of mass destruction and aimed at total victory or total defeat do not allow for the assessment of the relativity between means and ends. The empirical description of these historical experiences may differentiate and bring out shades of ambiguity in this judgment.

These lessons have not prevented wars from being fought in other places and in other political and geopolitical conditions up to the present.[7] At the same time, awareness has grown that conflicts and injustices do exist in the world in proportions—or, even better, in disproportions—that exceed warlike conflicts in their extent and that cannot be solved by violent solutions.[8] In such situations the just-war doctrine, it seems, tends toward a means of action no longer adequately covered by its ends, namely a "just order of peace." The credibility of a just-war concept is therefore questionable.

In the current debate on nuclear armaments, this problem has become more acute in view of the fact that a nuclear war may one day be waged. The area to which most questions are directed is the problem of proportionality. A major nuclear war would destroy friend and foe alike. The long-term consequences for life on earth are both unforeseeable and incalculable. As such they cannot be the subject of a "responsible" balancing of ends and means.

Extending this debate further into the ethical and legal claims of the just-war doctrine, and having put aside the many controversial and contradictory estimates of all the empirical factors of weapon technology, we see two dominant aspects: the use of weapons and the consequences. As mentioned above, the point in the debate of nuclear deterrence concerns the proportionality of the means to any conceivable war aim. In this respect, the discussion is developing in the direction of demands which would make it possible to limit a war and keep it in bounds. It is on these criteria that the demand for purely defensive weapons is based, a demand that is oriented toward defense as the only *justa causa*. Based on similar criteria is the demand to lessen our dependence on nuclear weapons or to get rid of them completely in favor of the so-called conventional weapons, which would then allow the waging of war according to the old conceptions of conventional war. The ethical constraint behind both sets of demands is unmistakable and is based on experience. However, in renewing the old concept of a just war (i.e., the revival of the *jus ad bellum* and *jus in bello* purely by means of a change of weapons), this ethical constraint is pointing in the wrong direction, namely into the past—when attempts were made to include war in the calculation for peace.

A further point concerns the relation between a possible use of nuclear weapons in an East-West conflict and the actual deployment of nuclear weapons within the deterrence strategy framework aimed at preventing such a war. The argument to be discussed here comes from the arsenal of arguments of the just-war doctrine, namely that those who deploy nuclear weapons must also be prepared, if necessary, to use them. This argument, when seen in the context of just-war doctrine, touches upon the *intentio recta* which, expressed in the language of moral theory, is the distinction between deployment and morally legitimate use. Although the deployment of nuclear weapons is primarily intended (*intentio recta*) to prevent war, paradoxically there must always be a readiness to use them. This paradox is both unavoidable and inevitable.

This argument has been put forward by the U.S. bishops regarding the just-war doctrine.[9] It is quite plainly an ethical dilemma. Germans who have joined the ranks of those involved in the above-mentioned conflict have referred to and, indeed, are concentrating on this line of argument, although they express it in a different way. However, this dilemma has, in principle at least, no solution.

Upon that basis, can an ethical demand for peace be made? The real perplexity here lies in the question of the actual "conditions of peace." In present-day discussion, talk of merely surviving has come to the fore. This ought to act as a signal for Christian peace ethics, the purpose of which consists of more than the mere amplification of perplexities and fears. Christian peace ethics should try to remove the spell that the sight of weapons of war is able to cast over our thinking.

The Crisis of the Concept of Peace[10]

Behind the ethical dilemma of nuclear deterrence another problem arises that is of even greater import. The traditional just-war doctrine arose from the framework of a "Peace Order Concept," obliging all partners in a conflict and relating them to each other. The criteria of a just war referred to this concept of peace. The idea of a "peace of God" (the medieval "Gottesfrieden") and that of justice, which was equally binding for all parties, served as an explicit, fundamental basis for all the parties in a conflict. That was also true for the modern community of sovereign states founded on common principles of law.

As a result of the revolutions of the late eighteenth century, the content and the efficiency of such a concept of peace have suffered a severe crisis. Most significantly, the previously unknown concept of the "war against the state" (i.e., the struggle against a certain form and constitution of the state, which must be overcome) has become a new reason for conflict and has a twofold consequence for the concept of peace still existing today.

War fought with the aim of a different political order is, then, no longer related to a common, universal order of peace embracing the conflicting parties and so limiting the conflict. Such a war seeks to destroy the false, antiquated, unlawful, or oppressive political order. It is no longer regulated by a given order of peace. Rather, the aim of war is to establish afresh the true order of peace. However, when the aim of war and the aim of peace are one and the same, then war itself can be construed as a promoter and source of future peace. To this extent, peace loses its normative regulatory power.

This leads us to the second consequence, namely that war in this sense can appear to be absolutely just because it is in principle the "war against war," i.e., the war against the real cause of previous wars which lies in the oppressive order to be overthrown. The war to end all wars has on its side the pathos of the last war. Secular messianic claims to the real peace are brought into play, and a claim of final peace takes precedence over any idea of an order of peace embracing the conflicts going on in the world.

The consequences of this development are all too easily recognizable: destruction followed by re-creation, but on a different basis. Peace is threatened far less by the weapons held in the hands of men than by the disagreement in convictions and the unreconciled conceptions of peace which no longer unite, but divide. This leads to the concepts of peace that have war as a necessary prerequisite. The concept of a uniting and obligating peace has reached a point of crisis, and herein lies the future real and decisive threat. Our era will be determined by this crisis; thus, any intellectual account of peace ethics must address it.

From the Doctrine of Just War to the Doctrine of Just Peace[11]

Thinking Toward Peace

What are the peace aims from which our actions should be derived, judged, and determined? This is the question presented by the just-war doctrine's basic ethical intent. Approached constructively, the legal and ethical meaning of this doctrine was to subject war, as a violent way of settling conflicts, to the concepts and the rule of law and justice, which themselves are supposed to be instruments of peace. The fundamental attitude to which the just-war doctrine appealed was, in short, thinking from the basis of peace! We are living in an era in which this appeal is being fundamentally questioned. That is true in the sharpest and most obtrusive way, especially with respect to the East-West conflict, which dominates all others.

The crisis of the concept of peace that marks our era did not start with the East-West conflict or with nuclear deterrence. The birth of modern pacifism, which has had its advocates in Europe since the last part of the nineteenth century, is itself a reaction to and a reflection of the power politics of antagonists no longer supported by a convincing concept of peace. Power politics is now reaching fruition under the influence of constant ideological tensions in the East-West conflict.

The profound questioning of the concept of peace itself encompasses the questioning of all the other peace-related criteria and orientations and thus involves political action as well as ethical consciousness. The fundamentals of law, justice, and responsibility lack the perspective to serve as more than a precarious management of a status quo that is missing in peace. To this extent, the role of weapons in the discussion has been that of a questionable substitute and representative for the image and concept of peace. Expectations and hopes of peace are being addressed to weapons, though these expectations hardly seem attainable by means of weapons, armament, or disarmament. If one considers the whole spectrum of moral, legal, philosophical, and political concerns, and if one equally regards the fullness of intellectual and spiritual resources put into this debate, then the objective lack of peace perspectives from which this era is suffering stands out all too plainly.

Therefore, if there is a task that can be grasped in moral and intellectual categories, then it is this: thinking toward peace.

The Concept of Peace

Nobody today would readily want to don the mantle of a new Augustine. But it might be helpful to discuss the cut and pattern of such a garment. If we could succeed in diverting to this task even a small part of the moral and intellectual energies which today are expended on the discussion of weapons and strategies, we would achieve a step in the right direction.

For Christians and for the churches alike, peace symbolizes, most importantly, the perspective of the peace of God as it appears in the Old Testament language of prophecy and promise and in the New Testament language of fulfillment and expectation. The message that we hear there, in secular measure, is that we live from peace and not from war. The same is also true in an ontological and ethical sense of human political and social life. The ethics of peace will have to ask what is to be gained from the images of universal reconciliation and all-sufficient fulfillment for a world which is anything but united in its beliefs and expectations and which cannot rely on the faith of Christianity as an enforceable condition for peace. Thus, the question arises as to how the expectation of peace can be translated into a task of peace toward which we can think.

A comparison might be helpful at this point. The World Health Organization has defined health in a way which—*mutatis mutandis*—might also be characteristic of an exacting peace concept. According to this definition, health is the state of complete physical, mental, and social well-being. The formula is an advance in medicine in that it revises the idea that health exists if one is free from bodily disturbances. Analogously, one can define peace (looking at political peace in particular) as being more than the absence of the immediate violence of war. In the complete sense, peace is a life which satisfies all, which brings peace in unclouded unanimity with oneself and one's neighbor, with the community of nations as a whole.

The logical conclusion from such a concept of peace can only be this: there is no peace in the world; furthermore, peace transcends the possibilities and capabilities of humanity. As purely a demand for what should be, such a concept of peace would tend to have more of a disorienting than an orienting function for the ethics of peace. The definition of health by the World Health Organization also leads us to the conclusion that nobody is healthy. Borrowing once again from this concept of health, we can maintain that health, rather than being the absence of disturbances, is the strength to cope independently with these disturbances and to live with them.[12] Transposing this concept onto the concept of peace, we can say, therefore, that peace is not the complete absence of political conflicts but is the sum of the abilities and instruments for dealing with them in something other than a violent manner. Peace is the ability to deal with conflicts politically. An active willingness for peace must live up to its political task. Peace is not the possession and exclusive claim of one system above or against another system, and therefore claims that peace results from the success of the international class struggle or that peace can be the victory only of democracy are false.[13] Rather, peace is a condition of the conflict of systems itself and demands a recognition that challenges the antagonistic aims of peace.

The Role of Military Force

Considering peace from this perspective, we must question anew the role of military force. As early as 1945 (i.e., long before nuclear deterrence had taken shape) Bernard Brodie had formulated the thesis that in the future, military armaments could be used only to prevent war.[14] Taking this a step further, and using a phrase that is completely opposite in its general direction, we can formulate the thesis: "Create peace without using weapons." The renunciation of force in international law, as formulated in the Kellogg-Briand Pact outlawing war as a means of pursuing and attaining political aims, assigns military power a limited role. The only rational and ethically comprehensible function of military force raised to the height of nuclear weapons is to make the renunciation of force compelling and to give this renunciation and its ethical, political, and legal demands an unavoidable and compelling instrument. At this point, military force can no longer be part of a just-war concept. This compelling renunciation of war is the imperative of nuclear deterrence in a world situation in which apparently antagonistic peace aims cannot otherwise be prevented from being realized. The existence and the escalation of nuclear deterrence are not the root, but the consequence, of this antagonism. Military force has, therefore, the task of compelling an antagonistic partnership of the systems.

Nuclear deterrence takes part in the perplexity of peace. It cannot be expected that the military guarantor of the prevention of war as such will also be the guarantor of a new concept of peace that will change this antagonism. The discussion about more or fewer weapons and armaments and about strategic planning is certainly not yet a peace debate. Indeed the movements which owe their existence to this discussion are still not yet adequate peace movements. The weight that nuclear weapons have thrown onto the scale of peace, the weight of the compelling renunciation of force, cannot and must not be reduced until we have succeeded in compensating for the weight of the antagonism of the systems by finding a concept of peace that embraces this antagonism and is able to change it.

Until that has been achieved, the function of military force, directed toward the renunciation of force altogether, will not be able to do away with the dilemma facing us. There are many difficult and delicate questions, of varying importance, as to how we can be pressured into renouncing force. This process must be well thought through and planned in advance in order to minimize, limit, and keep in bounds the use of force in case of an outbreak of military conflict. These questions and activities arise as a result of nuclear deterrence. However, not only ethical but also political and military reasons speak out strictly against ascribing to military planning a leading role as peacemaker. A just war is today no longer regarded as a means to a just peace. The prevention of war is the bond that links military power with the task of peace.[15]

The Problem of Peace in the Conflict of Systems

In order to measure the task with which we are confronted, we must take a good look at the historical roots of the conflict of systems that exist at this time. In its intellectual and spiritual roots the East–West conflict goes back well into the nineteenth century. Far from being just a military antagonism, it touches on almost all questions concerning the political and social constitution, the public estimate of culture and religion, and the relation of individual life and its rights to political society. Reconsidering clearly this conflict's history is an important requirement for all who want to extricate themselves from the spell of confrontation.

In addition to the renunciation of force (though we cannot as yet dispense with a military backup), there emerges the compulsion to coexist. In other words, the starting point for a new consideration of international justice is the recognition of interdependence. Justice by its very nature cannot be defined and realized one-sidedly; it should provide a form for a relationship of mutual dependence. What is true of economic justice is also true of political justice. Justice is, therefore, the opposite of the concept of domination of one over the other. Peace, as it has rightly been termed, is not a state or even a final state but a process. The questions with which we are faced today and which we must pose to our own discussion of peace are the following: (1) What change in the conflict of systems can we accelerate? and (2) How can such a transformation of the conflict of systems be set in motion or accelerated along already existing lines?

The imperative of change as a process of a new fashioning of peace is a political one, the perspective for which is to a large extent blocked by fences made of weapons, challenging us to look beyond them. The imperative of change cannot halt at a stability guaranteed by military confrontations, quite simply because this stability is not an adequate peace aim. One of the greatest and most significant elements of change is the conception of human rights,[16] the roots of which are to be found in an image of freedom. This freedom is, however, not identical with the boundaries and self-preserving interests of political systems, which are a law unto themselves. The concept of human rights is also founded upon a law prior and superior to every state, however it may be politically constituted. As for the perception and realization of human rights, we have no comparable means of compulsion available because human rights cannot, by their very nature, be based on compulsion. Their development and deployment as an inner yardstick for the change of political structures must therefore claim a freedom of movement, the conditions for which can be provided only by the state's monopoly of force.

But human rights do not merely exist as an idea or as a moral consciousness. They are closely connected with the economic, political, legal, and cultural organization of societies and systems. A change of systems that does not simply negate the maintenance of political systems or underestimate their importance must, therefore, be conceived as a process that makes it possible to approach the canon of human rights along material, economic, and organizational paths. Thus, the symmetry of a dogmatically oriented conception of human rights cannot determine the change either. In this perspective the thought of unilateralism (i.e., steps taken by one side) has the best chance of pointing to the future. Offers by the West to cooperate economically with the East—offers which are not tied to equally weighted or symmetrical performances by the East but which could help the independent evolution of still underdeveloped possibilities as a condition of more freedom of movement in the life of the East—could under certain circumstances be a suitable investment in the process of peace building. Although the Federal Republic of Germany's policies toward the East have sometimes been criticized because of their unbalanced unilateralism, they are a considerable contribution to such a transformation of the conflict of systems.

Internal and External Peace

What is true of the conflict of systems, namely that there is no military solution to it with a promise for the future, is also true "internally." It should never be forgotten that no society can in the long run be established on the foundation of military force alone. Protection from external force does not guarantee a just domestic peace. This aspect hardly plays a part in the tradition underlying the just-war doctrine, but it is nevertheless of great importance for us today. We are aware of the dangerous reactions which an external military confrontation taking place over a lengthy period of time—especially during times of peace—has upon the internal, moral, and juridical structure of our society. In principle, however, that is true for all nations.

One point that cannot be emphasized enough is that in a democracy there must be no mandate for self-destruction. Self-preservation of political power, however necessary it may be, cannot make use of any carte blanche. In the long run, therefore, the imperative of change must also be recognized as an imperative of political self-preservation. It is not at all cynical to say that high aims can be achieved only when they are allied with practical political interests.

The moral and political pressure on governments and majorities not to regard the existence of their own electors as hostage in a future war may not and should not be used without regard to constitutionally and legally regulated methods of political expression as to what they desire. This pressure and the movement that has resulted from it have so far produced no perspective which has taken us further in the direction of peace. However, it can still make the imperative of change in the peace process so compelling that its translation into political action does at least, out of the motives of political self-preservation, lead to new actions. Similarly, the unlimited discussion in free societies is a piece of unilateralism, in that possibilities and constraints of one-sided measures emerge which do not necessarily remain within the symmetry of the systems. The burden of freedom carries with it at this point the greater hope.

The Churches and Peace

The churches that today offer the peace discussion a forum entered this discussion in the fifth century with the just-war doctrine. They cannot simply extricate themselves from it on the basis that it does not fall within church affairs, nor can they do so on the basis that the whole direction of these modern problems in science, technology, and the conflict of systems is repugnant to them.

We are halfway between a just-war doctrine and a just-peace doctrine, and the churches have the important task of accompanying those who are along the way. Only if we have reason to hope that God has not abandoned the world and that God's peace holds sway over all we undertake, can we be encouraged to think toward peace. The churches cannot lay down a political perspective for peace, but it is their task to proclaim and assert that it is meaningful and not hopeless to engage in seeking a new peace perspective in and for the world.

Notes

1. Christian Walther, ed., *Atomwaffen und Ethik. Der deutsche Protestantismus und die atomare Aufrüstung 1954–1961. Dokumente und Kommentare* (München: Chr. Kaiser Verlag, 1981).

2. For the text of the Heidelberg Theses, see ibid.

3. See *Frieden wahren, fördern und erneuern. Eine Denkschrift der Evangelischen Kirche in Deutschland* (Gütersloh: Gütersloher Verlagshaus Gerd Mohn, 1981). In English, *The Preservation, Promotion and Renewal of Peace: A Memorandum of the Evangelical Church in Germany* (EKD Bulletin, 1982).

4. See *Gerechtigkeit schafft Frieden. Wort der Deutschen Bischofskonferenz zum Frieden,* 1983 (Schriftenreihe "Die deutschen Bischöfe" Nr. 34).

5. See *Das Bekenntnis zu Jesus Christus und die Friedensverantwortung der Kirche. Eine Erklärung des Moderamens des Reformierten Bundes* (Gütersloh: Gütersloher Verlagshaus Gerd Mohn, 1982).

6. See *Frieden stiften. Die Christen zur Abrustung. Eine Dokumentation. Herausgegeben und erlautert von Gunter Baadte, Armin Boyens und Ortwin Buchbender* (München: Verlag C. H. Beck, 1984). See also *Die Diskussion um die Friedensfrage in der Evangelischen Kirche in Deutschland, Kirchliches Jahrbuch,* 1983 (Gütersloh: Gütersloher Verlagshaus, 1985).

7. In the past thirty-five years there have been more than 140 wars with approximately ten million casualties. They have taken place beyond the bounds of nuclear deterrence. See Michael Quinlan, "Thinking Deterrence Through," in R. James Woolsey, ed., *Nuclear Arms: Ethics, Strategy, Politics* (San Francisco: ICS Press, 1984), 62.

8. This applies principally to the problems of developing countries and to the whole problem area of the North-South conflict. Nowadays it would be more appropriate to talk of the helplessness of war!

9. National Conference of Catholic Bishops, *The Challenge of Peace: God's Promise and Our Response* (Washington, D.C.: United States Catholic Conference, 1983). German translation in *Hirtenworte zu Krieg und Frieden* (Köln, 1983), 125–285. Concerning the discussions, see above all Albert Wohlstetter, "Bishops, Statesmen and Other Strategists on the Bombing of Innocents," *Commentary* 75 (1983): 15–35; and Albert Wohlstetter et al., "Morality and Deterrence," *Commentary* 76 (1983): 4ff. The German church statements make very little or no use of the just-war theory. See *Gerechtigkeit schafft Frieden,* in *Hirtenworte zu Krieg und Frieden* (Köln, 1983), and the German Protestant Church memorandum *Frieden wahren, fördern und erneuern.*

10. On the subject of the historical change in the concept of peace, see Wilhelm Janssen, "Frieden," in O. Brunner et al., *Geschichtliche Grundbegriffe. Historisches Lexikon zur politisch-sozialen Sprache in Deutschland,* vol. 2 (Stuttgart, 1975), 543–91.

11. This section develops the arguments that the just-war theory can no longer be applied in the nuclear age. The decisive turning point is the fact that there is no convincing ethical justification for a *jus ad bellum* in the event of a nuclear war. The North American debate has therefore concerned itself merely with *jus in bello* to gain ethical criteria for the use of atomic weapons. This quest for ethical criteria, as justified and necessary as it is, lacks the foundation as expounded in the *jus ad bellum* doctrine. An ethical and political peace doctrine must take its place. The aversion of nuclear war (deterrence) can provide an ethical and political foundation from which criteria for the use of nuclear weapons for deterrence or the ending of a nuclear war can be developed.

12. The argument here follows Dietrich Rössler, *Der Arzt zwischen Technik und Humanität* (München, 1977), 60–61.

13. See also Egbert Jahn, "Eine Kritik der sowjetisch-marxistischen Lehre vom 'gerechten' Krieg," in R. Steinweg, ed., *Der gerechte Krieg: Christentum, Islam, Marxismus* (Frankfurt, 1980), 163–85; and Gottfried Kiessling and Wolfgang Scheler, "Friedenskampf und politisch-moralische Wertung des Krieges," *Deutsche Zeitschrift für Philosophie* 24 (1976): 37–49.

14. Bernard Brodie et al., eds., *The Absolute Weapon: Atomic Power and World Order* (New York: Harcourt, Brace, 1946).

15. This point incorporates ideas from Klaus Ritter, "Einige Anmerkungen zur Friedensdiskussion," in *Frieden politisch fördern. Richtungsimpulse,* published by the Evangelische Kirche in Deutschland (Gütersloh, 1985), 11–32.

16. See, e.g., Jost Delbrück, "Menschenrechte: Grundlage des Friedens?" in Hans Thimme and Wilhelm Wöste, eds., *Im Dienst für Entwicklung und Frieden: In memoriam Bischof Heinrich Tenhumberg* (Mainz/München, 1982), 89–102.

III · THE CHURCHES

8 • Peacemaking as an Ethical Category: The Convergence of Pacifism and Just War

DUANE K. FRIESEN

The discipline of Christian ethics has inherited a time-honored tradition of categories for interpreting the differences between pacifism and just war from Ernst Troeltsch, the Niebuhrs, Roland Bainton, and others. These traditional typologies of sect-church and pacifism–just war impose themselves upon the debate as categories highlighting the polarities or tensions between the two traditions. James Johnson, in his recent book *The Quest for Peace,* continues this mode of thinking in summarizing the three positions explored in his book:

> Each of these perspectives generates its own myth of war, and each has its own concept of peace. Thus, not only do we find three traditions of the quest for peace flowing from these perspectives, we actually have three different goals that are all called by the same name: "peace." The peace of the sectarian community is the result of God's love, lived out in the common life by those who have received it. For those outside that love, there is no peace. The peace of just war tradition is the restraint of evil, which can never be completely stamped out but always threatens to break out anew. It is an interim state of life, hard won and precious to possess, but all too easy to see vanish again. The peace of the utopian tradition is the realization in human history of a moral ideal, the new political order of the community of humankind, in which justice will be done and violence and war will wither to nothingness. Absent the causes of war in disorder and injustice, there will be no war. Peace, then, is more than not having war: it is the final ideal that results from the prior achievement of two other ideals, right order and justice.

Johnson's own stance is that each of these positions is part of a larger whole. While each can draw something from the other, they simply view the world differently, and what each can learn from the other is that "one's own way of thinking is not the only possible one."[1]

My thesis is that a new way of thinking about war and peace is emerging in the contemporary situation which is bringing about a convergence between the just-war and pacifist positions. I shall refer to a number of recent statements by church leaders and scholars that make the claim that a new paradigm for thinking about war and peace is emerging. But before I proceed in my analysis, I would like to clarify what I mean and do *not* mean by convergence. *Webster's Third New International Dictionary* says that the word *converge* means "to tend toward one point: approach nearer together." The word *convergence* means the "tendency or movement toward union or uniformity." To converge does not mean that all differences have been removed. Significant differences remain between pacifism and just war. However, I will argue that the two positions are growing alike. Both positions approach issues of war and peace in a similar way despite their significant differences. These tendencies, I believe, are so significant that we can begin to talk about an emerging new paradigm for thinking about issues of war and peace.

The typological method, which has been the dominant methodology used by Christian ethicists for analyzing the ethical issue of war and peace, has several significant limitations preventing us from noticing areas of convergence.

1. It tends to rigidify the terms of the debate between positions, not sufficiently recognizing changes and movements in positions, or subtle differences within a particular position.
2. It tends to emphasize differences or oppositions between positions, not sufficiently recognizing points of commonality or convergence between positions.
3. Descriptive typologies often implicitly involve normative arguments, without this fact being made explicit by the persons using the typology.[2]
4. Typologies necessarily highlight the "essential" or central characteristics of a position. While this highlighting involves a tentative historical judgment subject to change, typologies tend to take on a permanence as if the categories of opposition between positions were metaphysically or eternally grounded.[3]

In this essay I will explore the fruitfulness of a methodology which seeks to identify commonly shared views between the two traditions of pacifism and just war. I will focus upon the ethical category of "peacemaking" as a central concept in both pacifist and just-war traditions to illuminate the convergence or significant shared commonality between the two traditions.[4] Both traditions share the deep concern about the potential threat of nuclear war to life as we know it. That concern alone has not brought about a significant change in the way just-war advocates and pacifists think theologically and ethically about war and peace. What that concern has done, however, is to shift the central question from whether or under what conditions the use of lethal force is legitimate to the question of how one prevents conflict from breaking out and how peace can be made between parties in conflict with each other.

Using just-war categories of thinking, many have concluded that a nuclear war cannot be justified under any circumstances. Francis X. Meehan's commentary upon the U.S. Catholic bishops' pastoral letter *The Challenge of Peace* is typical of this reasoning:

> The Church is moving and, I believe, must move to such a realistic evaluation of modern war that for all practical purposes it will become a Church of nonviolence. . . . Thus the just-war principles themselves, especially those of discriminacy and proportion, if we look at them closely and concretely, may help us to move to the necessity of a total rejection of war, and thus to a moral posture of nonviolence.[5]

The reasoning moves out of the categories of just-war thinking, but arrives at a position of practical pacifism that requires that the church's thinking be redirected to how to prevent war and make peace and away from the predominant question of the previous centuries: Under what conditions is war justified?

Here some might object that the just-war criterion of right intention has always had the pursuit of peace as its objective. That criterion, however, has been submerged in the tradition within the framework of the dominant question of the conditions under which war may be justified. The new emphasis turns the question upon its head: How can peace be made without resort to war? The new situation focuses our attention on the nonviolent means of conflict resolution, rather than directing our primary attention to the careful ethical discrimination which would justify the resort to war.

A shift in thinking has also occurred among pacifists that has led toward identification with some of the concerns that have been central in the just-war tradition. However, before I can identify those changes, I need to clarify which kind of pacifism I am talking about. One of the reasons for confusion in the current debate about war and peace is that persons are using the traditional categories of just war and pacifism without being clear how these terms are understood. I think the confusion is due particularly to the fact that very different understandings of pacifism are being used. Thus a discussion of commonalities or convergences between the two traditions cannot proceed without a definition of the pacifism that I will be comparing with the just-war tradition.

In his book *Nevertheless,* John Howard Yoder has identified over twenty different types of pacifism. For purposes of this essay I will analyze the relationship between just-war theory and one type of pacifism that I will label "evangelical pacifism." Though there are clearly other kinds of pacifism, I think it justified to select this type because it comes from a relatively coherent intellectual tradition currently focused in the writings of a number of persons within the academic community and the Society of Christian Ethics, the major professional society of Christian theological ethicists in North America. I refer to the work of Yoder, Stanley Hauerwas, Dale Brown, Ronald Sider, and others. I would place my own book *Christian Peacemaking and International Conflict* within this same tradition. I think these same emphases are found in groups like the Sojourner Community, or in the New Call to Peacemaking of the Historic Peace Churches.

Evangelical pacifism has the following central characteristics: It draws its fundamental definition from the Bible. This essentially means that the biblical concept of shalom (wholeness in all spheres of life) serves as an integrating concept both to describe God's redemptive activity in history and to describe the witness and mission of the church. Jesus Christ serves as the fundamental norm both for reflecting the nature of God and God's activity in history and for providing the model or norm for what it means to be fully human. Peacemaking is not an isolated or optional part of the Christian Gospel but is integral and central to Christian theological understanding.

The meaning of history for the Christian finds its locus in a new society —the church. Evangelical pacifism views the church as the primary locus where the reality of peacemaking must first of all find expression. The evangelical pacifist acknowledges a fundamental tension between the church, which seeks to embody the kingdom ethic of peacemaking in its life and practice, and the institutional structures of society, which are shaped primarily by the "realistic," by what is possible in a sinful world.

Nevertheless, the evangelical pacifist rejects withdrawal from the world. The church, both corporately and through individuals, is active in the world in giving witness to the possibility of shalom. It works actively to see shalom more adequately embodied in human social, political, and economic structures. This specifically means that the church is active in seeking to bring about justice for human social institutions and seeking to bring about nonviolent means of achieving justice both through the more normal processes of political and legal methods of nonviolent conflict resolution and through participation in the waging of nonviolent struggles for social change (in the Gandhi and Martin Luther King traditions). The activity of the church is carried out in the world in a broad arena of activity, such as helping give shape to the ethos of society, demonstrating justice and nonviolence through example, serving by organizing institutions to meet human need, seeking to influence and shape public policy, and working through vocations in public settings to foster shalom in all spheres of life.

While continuing to reason from a tradition of evangelical pacifism, persons within this stream of thought have begun to shift their attention from almost exclusive preoccupation with the theological basis for pacifism and its resultant ethical claim, the rejection of all violence, to concern with the question, How can justice be done and peacemaking be accomplished in a sinful world so that violence can be prevented? As is the case with just-war thinking, the central question is not whether violence is ever justified, but how peace can be preserved and how peace can be made when there is injustice and violence. To put it another way, the negative preoccupation of both just war and pacifism, whether violence can be justified, has shifted to a positive moral obligation, how peace can be made and preserved.

The Methodist bishops in their statement *In Defense of Creation* have sought to go beyond the pacifism–just-war debate by elaborating on areas where the two traditions converge, or where new issues and new approaches to the problems of war and peace simply transcend the traditional categories of debate. The Methodist bishops state this directly at several points in their document:

> We believe the nuclear crisis poses fundamental questions of faith that neither the pacifist nor just-war traditions have adequately addressed. We invite pacifists and nonpacifists among our people

not only to recapture their common ground, such as their moral presumption against all war and violence, but to undertake together a fresh inquiry into those transcendent issues that stretch far beyond private conscience and rational calculation. . . . In the roundedness of shalom, a just-war ethic is never enough. Our churches must nurture a new theology for a just peace.

Over the centuries three classical positions developed among Christian thinkers and church bodies: pacifism, "just-war" doctrine, and the crusade. While this threefold division never fully reflected the diversity of Christian views, it is particularly outmoded and inadequate for clarifying the ethical dilemmas of the nuclear arms race.

We confess that the churches' response to primal nuclear issues over the past four decades has been fitful and feeble. At the same time we recognize that some theologians in the first years after Hiroshima, and again in the 1980's, have earnestly sought to address these primal issues. Typically, they have drawn on pacifist and just-war traditions in their efforts. We are equally troubled by the inadequate response of churches and theologians to the consequent nuclear issues. These consequent issues stretch farthest beyond the classical war-peace debate. They cut most sharply into the systemic fabric of our cultural and institutional life. They make most clear that the nuclear crisis is an issue of social justice as well as world peace. And they make the wholeness of the shalom vision most imperative for our time.

As most denominations and ecumenical bodies have become freshly engaged in the nuclear debate since 1980, the classical threefold typology (pacifist/just-war/crusade) has proved increasingly inadequate to contain the burgeoning variety of ethical positions.[6]

These statements suggest that the bishops are groping for a way to describe an emerging paradigm. In the above statements and throughout their document they are making several claims that can be shared by both just war and pacifism: (1) the moral presumption against all war and violence; (2) the idolatry of embracing nuclear weapons systems as a basis for ultimate security; (3) the threat to social justice by the waste of so many human intellectual and economic resources on the arms race; and (4) the need to make peace, through a reciprocal process of gradual disarmament, the only lasting basis for security.

In developing a statement that goes beyond pacifism and just war, however, the Methodist bishops have created a position that at times seems incoherent and confused. Methodist theologians Paul Ramsey and

Stanley Hauerwas have pointed out this confusion. Despite this claim of the Methodist bishops to transcend the pacifist–just-war debate, Hauerwas argues that the bishops have obscured basic differences between the two traditions and that this has led to confusion in the document.

> I believe the bishops have not shown us that the issue of nuclear war requires the church to develop a position beyond just war or pacifism. Indeed I think they would have helped us be more faithful as Christians if they had challenged the church to think through both the common commitments and differences between the just war perspective and the pacifist.[7]

What the bishops failed to do was address the church unambiguously, helping to clarify the theological foundations of Christian peacemaking. In some respects the document does reflect a theological orientation rooted in the Scriptures and addressed to the church. They appeal to the authority of scriptural teaching, which leads them to the view that war is incompatible with the teachings and example of Christ. In several places in the document the bishops call for the church to be an alternative community. But instead of following this direction, the bishops have developed a position that is shaped *primarily* by a secular philosophy, the urgency to avoid nuclear destruction. The consequence of this starting point is confusion about to whom the pastoral letter is addressed. Because the bishops address governments who hold in their hands the power to destroy the earth, they cannot simply affirm pacifism. That would undermine the very existence of government, insofar as government rests on the availability of the sword to protect good and punish evil.

The bishops' ambivalence is also reflected in how they treat the issue of deterrence. Deterrence is contrary to pacifism, yet it cannot simply be abandoned, because governments must work toward disarmament through a reciprocal process over time. Thus deterrence is wrong from a Christian point of view because of its threat to genuine security, yet it cannot be abandoned by governments in the short run. Also, because the bishops seem to want to allow for the possibility of violence in liberation movements, they cannot affirm pacifism wholeheartedly.[8] The ambivalence about audience is above all reflected in their quotation from their Social Principles statement:

> We believe war is incompatible with the teachings and example of Christ. We therefore reject war as an instrument of national foreign

policy and insist that the first moral duty of all nations is to resolve by peaceful means every dispute that arises between or among them.[9]

The first statement about the authority of Jesus Christ for the church is joined with a "therefore" that directs how nations are to behave in foreign policy. So the bishops cannot quite affirm pacifism. Yet simply to adopt the just-war position would not describe the new direction in which they want to go.

Though the Methodist statement is incoherent and confused, nevertheless I believe the bishops are searching for a direction that does move toward a convergence of pacifist and just-war thinking in some important respects.

One can also observe in the Catholic bishops' statement an effort to draw upon insights from both pacifist and just-war traditions, although interpreters of their statement do not agree in what sense there has been a real movement beyond traditional categories. Darrell Schmidt argues that the pacifist content of the bishops' scriptural exegesis is not operative at the level of moral theory in the document as a whole, where just-war categories dominate.[10] The bishops seem to want a position that recognizes the validity of both a pacifist and a just-war position for Christians. However, this is possible by declaring that the church's corporate position is just war, whereas pacifism is an appropriate position only for individual Christians within the church.[11]

David Hollenbach believes that the pastoral letter's statement of the complementary relationship of pacifism and just war (par. 74) is a genuinely new element in Catholic teaching.

> The pastoral's position on the complementarity of the just-war ethic and ethic of non-violence had not been affirmed previously in these explicit terms in the conciliar and papal teaching since World War II. The United States bishops are aware that they are breaking new ground in affirming this interdependence of just-war and pacifist perspectives in the contemporary situation. The impetus for such development comes from the conditions of the "new moment" in which we are located—a moment characterized by the massive destructive potential of nuclear weapons and by the new public perception of the dangers of these weapons.[12]

That something genuinely new has emerged here is reflected by a critic of the pastoral letter. In his recent book *Tranquillitas Ordinis*, George Weigel argues that the bishops have abandoned the classic heritage. One part of the abandonment is "the letter's confusion on the compatibility of the just-war and pacifist traditions. . . . The pastoral letter's argument that just-war theory and pacifism were interdependent methods of evaluating warfare is, to put it plainly, false. . . . The confusion of these two positions leads to the corruption of both."[13] Weigel defines the difference at the level of moral theory this way: the pacifist opposes all use of armed force, whereas the just-war theorist allows the proportionate and discriminate use of force in carefully defined circumstances. Weigel, however, goes on to say that while the two positions are not reconcilable at the level of moral theory, the letter does not sufficiently illuminate possibilities of practical cooperation, for "there is no reason why pacifists and just-war theorists cannot work together in the practical order on building international political community sufficient to sustain legal and political means of resolving conflict."[14]

What is going on? Is pacifist and just-war thinking converging? We have seen that both Protestant and Catholic scholars do not agree. Are the statements of the Methodist and Catholic bishops simply confused and lacking coherence, or are the critics so bound up with traditional categories of analysis focusing upon areas of disagreement that they have failed to sufficiently note possible areas of commonality?

One of the major areas of confusion regards what kind of pacifism is being compared with just war. Given the description of evangelical pacifism outlined earlier, many of the traditional polarities distinguishing just war and pacifism are simply inappropriate. Some of these traditional ways in which pacifism and just war have been distinguished are the following:

peace vs. justice
utopianism vs. realism
perfectionism vs. the reality of sin
withdrawal vs. political involvement
ideal vs. the real
Christ vs. culture
otherworldly apocalyptic vs. theology of culture

What can we say about these traditional oppositions?

Peace and justice are not opposites. Rather, evangelical pacifism is an ethic concerned with and actively involved in working for justice as well as peace. Some thinkers, like Richard Mouw, would argue that there is ultimately a tension between pacifism and just war relating to peace and justice.

The ongoing debates between Christian pacifists and just war theorists can be viewed as an important argument over how we should
deal with this experienced tension, with one side arguing that in the
present dispensation the primary emphasis must be placed on a
consistently non-violent witness to the promise of peace, and the
other side insisting that the doing of justice requires us on occasion
to commit acts of violence.[15]

He believes that only in the Reign of Christ can and will peace and justice
unite.

I remain unconvinced by the argument that this distinguishes pacifism and just-war theory, for three reasons:

First, the tension between peace and justice exists within both just war
and pacifism, not between them. One should seek justice according to just-
war theory, but one may *not* do that if the means used to bring about justice
violate other standards like noncombatant immunity, proportionality, or
a reasonable chance of success. Thus justice does not always take
precedence over peace, but there is a tension between them. Similarly,
pacifists believe strongly in working for justice, but not if that violates
certain standards like restraints against violence to bring about justice.

Second, both positions also believe strongly in the interconnections
between peace and justice. Without justice there cannot be *stable* peace,
though the existence of justice is often not a *necessary* condition for avoiding war. Just-war theorists tend to emphasize this side of the equation.
The other side of the equation is that without peace, justice is unobtain-
able. Pacifists, such as Kenneth Boulding, tend to emphasize this side of
the equation:

Justice is most easily increased when there is a strong sense of community, when the "integrative systems," as I have called them, are
visible and strong. People then feel bonds of fellowship and empathy
with others, and the poverty of the poor is seen as a disgrace by the
rich. Another important condition for the increase in justice is that
the political structure should have a minimum degree of competence,
defined as the ability not only to want the right things but to know
what has to be done to get them.

War, whether international or internal, tends to destroy these pre-
conditions of the dynamics of increasing justice. It creates enemies
and enmities, it destroys the larger sense of community, it destroys
the sense of common humanity. In order to justify our own violence
we have to deny humanity to its victims. There is a fair amount of

evidence that the most just societies that we see around the world, that are accepted by their citizens as reasonably just without strong dissent, are those that have been created by the slow growth of the sense of community, that on the whole have abjured violence, that have believed in buying people off rather than knocking them down, and that have had reasonably competent government.[16]

Third and finally, at the theological level, it is because peace and justice are united in the Reign of God that they are united in the church's work in the world. The church is a community which trusts in God's kingdom as the ultimate reality governing its life in the world. As such, the church lives by its commitment to Jesus Christ, who brought healing (justice) to the world nonviolently. Evangelical pacifism is realistic about the sinful structures of the world and also about the problem of sin within the church (thus the concern for repentance and discipline in the church). The dichotomy between realism and utopianism, or perfectionism, is not fundamentally at issue between the two positions. Evangelical pacifism is also profoundly active in the world. The labels of withdrawal, Christ vs. culture, or an otherworldly apocalypticism are simply not applicable.

Thus it is not surprising to find the recognition by the Catholic and Methodist bishops of a certain convergence between pacifism and just war, a movement beyond the categories that have traditionally defined the difference between the two positions.

However, I think the key factor in this convergence is the influence of a common biblical theology of shalom, which has had a profound effect upon both just-war and pacifist traditions. One cannot help but be struck by the agreement among the Methodist bishops, Catholic bishops, and evangelical pacifists about the meaning and centrality of shalom in the Bible. Here I would give much more credit to the Methodist bishops than does Stanley Hauerwas. This common emphasis upon shalom has given shape to the following common emphases in both the just-war and pacifist traditions:

1. The centrality of justice to the shalom vision.
2. The linkage of shalom to God's redemptive activity in history. Shalom is integral to Christian theology.
3. The emphasis upon and preference for nonviolent means for seeking justice and resolving conflict.

4. The centrality of the church in giving witness to and embodying shalom. Though the Methodist bishops do not spell out the implications of their position, they refer on several occasions to the necessity of an alternative community to live out and give witness to the shalom vision.
5. The recognition of sin as it is expressed in nationalism, the idolatry involved in the trust in military power and weapons systems to provide security, and the violation of justice in the use of scarce human resources for an arms race that inevitably robs the poor.

At a more practical level there is common agreement:

1. Nuclear weapons must never be used.
2. Criticism of deterrence grows, though the Catholic and Methodist bishops and evangelical pacifists do not agree about whether deterrence may still be a short-run necessity.
3. Interest grows in the development of strategies and techniques of nonviolent conflict resolution, and in the development of international structures that can provide a peaceful alternative to solving conflict with arms.
4. The development of particular types of weapons systems is dangerous because of the increased insecurity and the increased danger of nuclear war they are likely to bring.

This list of commonalities between the two positions is not exhaustive, but it is sufficient to point out very significant convergences. Convergence does not mean agreement. But having focused our thinking more clearly upon areas of convergence, we can more accurately identify the real issues still at stake in the debate.

George Weigel, referring to an article by James Finn, argues that pacifism and just war are fundamentally incompatible at the level of moral theory: "The principled pacifist opposes all resort to armed force; the just-war theorist allows the proportionate and discriminate use of armed force in carefully defined circumstances."[17] While this is true, I do not believe this point identifies the fundamental tension between pacifism and just war. It seems to me that the tension between the two positions is rooted in a basic theological polarity characteristic of the Christian faith and thus is a polarity that *all* Christians must struggle with. This is the tension between the kingdom of God—God's rule and sovereignty over the entire creation, which in some sense has "already" come—and the reality of a sinful world "not yet" transformed into the kingdom of God. The tension between the "already" and the "not yet" must be struggled with by every Christian, by every theological position. Pacifism tends to emphasize the "already" side of the polarity. It urges that Christians within an alternative community live out the new reality of God's peace and seek to give witness to that new reality in a sinful world. Just war tends to emphasize the "not yet" side of the polarity. It recognizes the need for force in a world of sin where God's kingdom has not been fully realized. But each must recognize the truth of the other: pacifism the reality of sin, just war the reality of God's kingdom which has broken into history in Jesus Christ. Thus the underlying truth of the two positions is a polarity that both recognize. In this sense pacifism and just war represent "complementary" truths in the Christian church, rather than positions that are necessarily opposites. Perhaps an analogy to the analysis of light in physics can illumine this issue. From one perspective light appears as a wave, from another as a particle. Ian Barbour describes the principle of complementarity this way:

> Most physicists . . . would probably subscribe to (Niels) Bohr's advice: retain both wave and particle models but recognize their limitations. "A complete elucidation of one and the same object," Bohr writes, "may require diverse points of view which defy a unique description." (Niels Bohr, *Atomic Theory and the Description of Nature*, p. 96) A duality of representation is required, since differing aspects of the structure of events are interpretable by differing models, each of which is incomplete and applicable only to certain experimental situations.[18]

Barbour's description recognizes two realities that apply to the pacifist–just-war debate. Both must recognize their limitations, and each is required—or, more accurately, both together are required—to interpret reality. It is the differing theological emphasis in the "already" and "not yet" polarity that leads to differences at the level of moral theory.

The fundamental tension is also expressed in two different interpretations of history.[19] We have two different visions of the future. One of these visions believes that our life in this world (i.e., the peace in the earthly city) is secured through the nation-state. From the point of view of the nation-state, war always remains a possibility. Thus the Catholic bishops hold that defense of the nation-state justifies the use of armed force. In a world of sin, nations must have the right to defend themselves against unjust attack, and thus war must always be a possibility. The evangelical pacifist trusts ultimately that the kingdom of God is present in Jesus Christ and is above all embodied in the earthly city in the new community—the church. Christian pacifism views history from the standpoint of God's kingdom, which has already broken into history in Jesus Christ and which has made possible a reconciliation and peace between people who are normally hostile to each other. The church is called to live out this history within the present reality. Thus the difference between the two positions ultimately involves a tension between how one understands the "already" represented by the church and the "not yet" represented by the state.[20]

I think it highly significant that the Catholic bishops use the language of a "complementary relationship" between pacifism and just war.[21] I was thus pleased to discover that Francis X. Meehan, in interpreting the bishops' statement, had arrived at a point of view similar to my own—the complementarity of just war and pacifism:

> Our protest against the increasing militarization must be sustained and vigorous, must pervade the whole Church, its structures, and its grass-roots organizations. This can happen only when there is some pull from an eschatological kingdom, some sense of grace, some awareness that force is an element of concupiscence which stems from sin, and which therefore must be moderated, diminished, progressively abolished. This kind of theological rooting of just-war teaching will put us in sympathetic dialogue with the pacifist who insists on total nonviolence. No longer will we see them in opposition, but rather only in tension. . . . Once we put just-war teaching in the context of a theology of sin and grace, we see how a new doctrine can develop in continuity with the old, and how there can be a progressive movement in the Church toward nonviolence, and finally how the two are not dichotomous but "complementary" realities.[22]

Similarly, from the point of view of evangelical pacifism we can see a movement to recognize the issues raised by the just-war perspective. I refer here to my own position in *Christian Peacemaking and International Conflict,* a position that I believe is representative of the development of thinking in a number of evangelical pacifists.

> [Christian] peacemaking must be extended to work for those overall conditions of society and the physical environment which can lead to a full and holistic human development for all persons. . . . In order

for Christians to relate their theological perspective effectively to the human situation, they must be able to translate the theological-ethical norms that are meaningful within the community of faith into principles that are applicable to the political order. This translation process is necessary in order to bridge two gaps: the gap between the more particular community of faith and the larger political community, and the gap between the church and political institutions. Some would argue that there is a necessary conflict between political institutions and the church, because the essence of politics is the "sword," i.e. the ultimate sanction is violent force. Though violent force is present in political institutions, political institutions cannot be reduced to this definition, as if violent force were necessary for political institutions to remain political. The essential purpose of political institutions is cooperation for the sake of the common good. Coercive violence is often not operative. We tend to exaggerate its importance.[23]

Because the Christian pacifist starts from the point of view that it is possible within history to trust in the reality of the kingdom of God, he or she believes that God's work in the world is most effective in a community of peace and nonviolence, not in the nation-state where resort to armed force is a constant possibility. As a public citizen the Christian pacifist contributes to the well-being of the society by working toward the achievement of justice through nonviolent means of change. The Christian pacifist is actively involved in the world to help develop an alternative to war and establish alternative systems of dispute settlement. Though this vision must be balanced with an awareness that is realistic about the tragic situations in which nations are caught, the institution of warfare is not seen as inevitable, because the evangelical pacifist operates also from the perspective of an eschatology which sees the triumph of the Lamb as the dominant power in history.

Nevertheless, evangelical pacifism might relate to a world where the sword is operative. I will choose one very complex and tough issue to illustrate the method the evangelical pacifist must use to make the transition from the church to the political realm. The question of how the Soviet Union and the United States can extricate themselves from the instability of deterrence is an appropriate issue for intellectual analysis and practical action by the evangelical pacifist. Both the Methodist and the Catholic bishops also seek to address this problem realistically.[24] That they seek to do so is not at issue for the evangelical pacifist. Insofar as the evangelical pacifist also seeks to address the well-being of society as a whole, he or she can agree with the recognition by the Methodist and Catholic bishops that the movement away from deterrence must be a step-by-step process. The evangelical pacifist too must imaginatively translate the shalom vision into realistic alternatives that can lead toward shalom within the political order. In fact, the evangelical pacifist can even appropriately employ just-war categories as a set of middle axioms to judge the behavior of nations when they are unable or unwilling to abandon trust in armed force as the way to peace. Within the political realm, the Christian pacifist can cooperate with the just-war advocate in calling for nations to abide by standards of just war.

That both the Catholic and the Methodist bishops cannot accept deterrence in the long run is their implicit recognition of the centrality of the church and its shalom vision. It is ultimately unacceptable for Christians to threaten to do violence against others in order to deter them from violence. Christians cannot simultaneously proclaim the good news of the Gospel and threaten their Soviet brothers and sisters with nuclear war. The Catholic bishops have recognized this contradiction both at the level of shalom and at the level of just-war theory. At the level of just-war theory, one cannot simultaneously forbid all use of nuclear weapons and have a credible deterrent, where one's opponent believes that one intends to use the weapons. In connection with their critique of deterrence the Methodist bishops have also called for the church to stand as an alternative community in the world.

The problem for evangelical pacifists, and the Methodist and Catholic bishops, is how to preserve the integrity of the church and at the same time speak realistically to the political realm. As an address to the church, the evangelical pacifists and just-war advocates appropriately call for an alternative community, for an alternative to the violent and unstable ethic of mutually assured destruction. As an address to the political community, the documents appropriately call for a realistic step-by-step process of movement away from deterrence. The problem for both pacifism and the just-war position is to avoid confusion about which audience one is addressing. From the point of view of the "already" realized kingdom, an alternative way of peace is possible in an alternative community—the church. Once we are clear about that possibility, we can address the "not yet," the issues of war and peace at the political level. At the political level, from the perspective of the church's shalom vision, the church can then appropriately assess and give support to those specific government policies that move in a direction that will eventually make deterrence obsolete. Within this sphere, a step-by-step process must be imagined and acted upon.

We can say that there are differences and crucial issues distinguishing just war and pacifism, though these tensions or polarities are not adequately identified by traditional typologies. One way we can treat these differences is simply to accept the fact that there are differences among Christians, that no one position can contain the whole truth, and that each needs the other to correct its own inadequacies. This perspective has, at its best, recognized that truth is greater than any one of the particular positions. On the negative side, this kind of thinking has led to a type of relativism, where the agreement to accept diversity has led to a lack of engagement about the truth claims of differing traditions, and a lack of real encounter at the level of theological and moral argument. The areas of convergence and commonality between the two positions suggest, however, a much more important fact. Christians do share a common identity shaped by the memory of Jesus Christ and embodied in the one holy Catholic Church. The common norm of Christian peacemaking is increasingly leading to areas of convergence and agreement between the just-war and pacifist traditions. This suggests that we go beyond our traditional propensity simply to agree to differ, that we continue to search for and find in each other that common truth which we have in Jesus Christ.

Notes

1. James Turner Johnson, *The Quest for Peace: Three Moral Traditions in Western Cultural History* (Princeton: Princeton University Press, 1987), 282–83.

2. Typologies function both as descriptive models to illuminate the past and as prescriptions about how to conceive of the contemporary options confronting Christians. I have shown elsewhere how Troeltsch is not interested only in descriptive sociology (and this distinguishes his use of typology from Max Weber's). His historical and sociological analysis is also intended to help solve the normative problem for the modern world. Troeltsch hopes to draw conclusions about what "ought to be" from his description of what is happening in history. (See my dissertation, "The Relationship Between Ernst Troeltsch's Theory of Religion and His Typology of Religious Association," Harvard University, 1972; and my essay entitled, "A Critical Analysis of Troeltsch's Typology of Religious Association," to appear in a collection of essays on Troeltsch published by Andrew Mellon Press.) Typologies are not value neutral, but they usually reflect the connection being made between the past and the present, what can be learned from the past to give guidance in the future. Troeltsch's *Social Teachings,* while a description of options in church history, is also implicitly an argument for the church type. H. R. Niebuhr's *Christ*

and Culture is not a neutral description of five types but is implicitly an argument why the fifth type, Christ the transformer of culture, is more adequate than the other types. In this sense the typology serves to describe that history with which the historian identifies and which he believes should be sustained and that type which is flawed in the past and should be rejected in the present. The weight of these typologies continues, thus, to shape the logic of ethical debate in the present.

3. Typologies are imaginative constructions by the modern historian which seek to illuminate the past by highlighting the options available to the actors. This means that these constructions are subject to revision, for they do not exist in immediately obvious form in the documents themselves. The modern historian must make a judgment about what the central categories are which distinguish a position. The historian also must judge which documents to select as "typifying" a particular position. For example, Johnson selects the Anabaptist *Schleitheim Confession of Faith* as typifying sectarian pacifism, a position which reinforces the Troeltschian characterization of the sect-type as withdrawal from the world. I am quite convinced, for example, that the portrayal of the sixteenth-century pacifist ethic of the Anabaptists as withdrawal from the world is fundamentally mistaken. Though I cannot engage in that historical analysis here, a fully developed position would draw upon modern historiography, which has recognized that the Anabaptist movement is diverse with respect to political involvement and that Schleitheim is only one option among several and does not describe the essence of the movement more than others. For example, Menno Simons gave ethical admonition to magistrates. The original vision of the followers of Zwingli in Zurich involved a call for a total social transformation. Withdrawal came only after persecution. Pilgrim Marpeck worked as a city engineer in Strasbourg and elsewhere and did not rule out political involvement by Christians. Some Anabaptists were clearly influenced by the general concern for social justice that was part of the peasants' revolution of the sixteenth century. Others even tried to set up a new utopian society (i.e., Münster). Thus when the traditional typology portrays the two positions of just war and pacifism as political involvement vs. withdrawal, the point of divergence between the two positions is fundamentally distorted, areas of commonality between the two positions are obscured, and the real differences between pacifism and just war are not illuminated. For the recent changes in historiography on the Anabaptist movement, see James Stayer, "The Anabaptists," in Steven Ozment, ed., *Reformation Europe: A Guide to Research* (St. Louis: Center for Reformation Research, 1982), 135–60; and Abraham Friesen, "Social Revolution or Religious Reform? Some Salient Aspects of Anabaptist Historiography," in Hans-Jurgen Goertz, ed., *Umstrittenes Taufertum 1525–1975* (Göttingen: Vandenhoeck and Ruprecht, 1975).

4. Richard Mouw, for example, after describing areas where pacifists and just-war defenders disagree, goes on to identify peacemaking and the development of a peace theology as areas of common commitment shared by pacifists and just-war theorists. Mouw, "Christianity and Pacifism," in *Faith and Philosophy* 2, no. 2 (April 1985): 105–11.

5. Francis X. Meehan, "Nonviolence and the Bishops' Pastoral: A Case for the Development of Doctrine," in Judith A. Dwyer, ed., *The Catholic Bishops and Nuclear War* (Washington, D.C.: Georgetown University Press, 1984).

6. United Methodist Council of Bishops, *In Defense of Creation: The Nuclear Crisis and a Just Peace* (Nashville, Tenn.: Graded Press, 1986).

7. Stanley Hauerwas, "A Pacifist Response to *In Defense of Creation,*" *Asbury Theological Journal* 41, no. 2 (Fall 1986): 14.

8. *In Defense of Creation*, 26–27.

9. Ibid., 20.

10. Darrell Schmidt, "The Biblical Hermeneutics on Peacemaking in the Bishops' Pastoral," *Biblical Theology Bulletin* 16, no. 2 (April 1986): 46–55.

11. Stanley Hauerwas, *Against the Nations: War and Survival in a Liberal Society* (Minneapolis: Winston Press, 1985), 189.

12. David Hollenbach, "*The Challenge of Peace* in the Context of Recent Church Teachings," in Philip J. Murnion, ed., *Catholics and Nuclear War: A Commentary on "The Challenge of Peace"* (New York: Crossroad, 1983), 6–7.

13. George Weigel, *Tranquillitas Ordinis: The Present Failure and Future Promise of American Catholic Thought on War and Peace* (Oxford: Oxford University Press, 1987), 283.

14. Ibid.

15. Mouw, "Christianity and Pacifism," 105.

16. Boulding goes on to cite evidence for his position: "It was not Oliver Cromwell but the 'Glorious Revolution' of 1688, in which not a shot was fired, which set Britain off on a path to greater riches and justice. The Meiji Restoration in Japan in 1868 was rather similar. Australia and Canada internally are much more peaceable and relaxed societies than the United States. Neither of them had a revolution or a civil war, although their tie-in with the British Empire involved them in some very traumatic foreign wars, such as World War I and II, from which the independence of the United States did not save it either. The French Revolution produced Napoleon, Oliver Cromwell produced the tragedy of Ireland, the Russian Revolution produced Stalin. There may be exceptions to this rule, but they are hard to find. The appeal to justice is often disguised self-justification. A just war is one that is easily justified, no matter what the evidence to the contrary." Kenneth Boulding, "Peace, Justice, Freedom, and Competence," *Zygon* 21, no. 4 (December 1986): 526–27.

17. Weigel, *Tranquillitas Ordinis,* 283.

18. Ian G. Barbour, *Issues in Science and Religion* (New York: Harper and Row, 1966), 290–91.

19. Hauerwas, *Against the Nations,* 195.

20. This difference in emphasis is illustrated by Mouw, who begins his explanation of why he is not a pacifist by emphasizing the role of government when it comes to the maintenance of peace in the world: "Many of us are not pacifists. We believe that governments have been invested by God with the legitimate authority to use the sword in both the internal policing of the affairs of nations and in the defense of nations against external enemies. We also believe that there are circumstances in which citizens are justified in wielding the sword against their own governments, when those governments have become agents of systematic oppression. Furthermore, we believe that it is permissible—perhaps even obligatory on occasion—for Christian citizens to participate in these violent activities." Mouw, "Christianity and Pacifism," 105. Though Mouw does not refer here to Romans 13, I suspect further debate would turn to the interpretation of that passage. The evangelical pacifist would claim that the perspective Paul is writing from is that of an adviser of the *church:* advising Christians to live nonviolently (ch. 12) but nevertheless to have proper respect for the semblance of order in the world provided by the state.

21. National Conference of Catholic Bishops, *The Challenge of Peace: God's Promise and Our Response* (Washington, D.C.: United States Catholic Conference, 1983).

22. Meehan, "Nonviolence," 100.

23. Duane K. Friesen, *Christian Peacemaking and International Conflict: A Realist Pacifist Perspective* (Scottdale, Pa.: Herald Press, 1986), 105.

24. A realist is one who understands the world the way it is. Boulding puts it this way: "Realism is some kind of more or less accurate mapping between the image of the world in the decision maker's head and the real world that lies in and around it. Competence,

therefore, always involves a learning process by which experience leads to a diminution in error. Error has two aspects: there may be error in the image of the environment around us— we may believe things about the world that are not true—or there may be error in the evaluation system by which we evaluate alternative futures leading us into decision which we or others eventually regret." Boulding, "Peace, Justice, Freedom, and Competence," 531. Realism should be common to both traditions. Both pacifist and just-war theorists are constantly testing each other in terms of the "realism" of each other's position. Just-war theorists often exaggerate the place of war and romanticize its positive effects. Pacifists tend to overlook the prevalence of violence and the difficulties of achieving justice nonviolently. I cannot here discuss the complex issues surrounding deterrence, but I chose this issue because it is one of the most difficult and complex issues of political judgment and thus can illustrate the method by which a Christian pacifist relates Christian ethics to politics. See the realism brought to bear on this issue in Alan Geyer, *The Idea of Disarmament!* (Elgin, Ill.: Brethren Press, 1982), 27–59; and also the helpful analysis of the moral arguments in and around the Catholic bishops' statement in David Hollenbach, S.J., *Nuclear Ethics: A Christian Moral Argument* (New York: Paulist Press, 1983), 63–85.

9 · Reason and Authority in Church Social Documents: The Case for Plausibility and Coherence

TODD WHITMORE

> What Epicurus called Necessity, Vico called Providence; what Kant called the Plan of Nature, Hegel called the Cunning of Reason. Yet, whether one entitled the agent of destiny Reason or Nature, Providence or Necessity, the practical significance of this doctrine was the same. No judgement on Man's success in the rational organization of his experience is ever final, or immune from reconsideration. However much we may seem to have achieved—however much we may *actually* have achieved—future problem-situations may always impose unforeseeable demands on our procedures, techniques and methods of thought.
>
> STEPHEN TOULMIN[1]

My task is to argue that the complex nature of modern public life in general and the problem-situation of the possession and potential use of nuclear weapons in particular require religious institutions to reconsider their understanding of the reason and authority of their social documents. This shall be done in three parts. The first section is primarily descriptive: it sets out the first option in the Roman Catholic tradition, what I term the "deductive-official" model. It is a model marked by a concern with the certainty, immutability, and universality of its claims and the status of the officeholders who make them. Once the general principles are issued from a recognized office, logical entailment is the criterion of the adequacy of specific judgments. The second section moves from description to construction in elaborating an alternative, the "responsive-magisterial" approach, which aims for the perdurability and continuity of a community's response over time to varying problem-situations. The criteria are the plausibility and coherence of the response as a whole. Thus my subtitle. Part three is primarily evaluative, and argues that the responsive-magisterial model is more adequate to address issues of consequence to human social life.

Underpinning this argument is the observation that method (mode of reasoning) and ecclesiology (understanding of authority) are linked. This is so because they constitute two dimensions—the conceptual and the organizational—of the activity or practice of a community as it seeks to address issues of consequence. Alterations in one dimension affect the other as well. As will be shown, the ultimate reason that the deductive-official model is inadequate is that it was originally intended to guide a quite different kind of activity than that involved in large social issues. It primarily aided priests in the sacrament of penance. The locus and scope of practice have since changed. So must the understanding of reason and authority.

My focus will be on the Roman Catholic case because, in general, its tradition of reason and authority is more developed than is the case in Protestant documents. It also needs to be noted that under consideration is a Roman Catholic case of a particular kind: a social document issued by a bishops' conference. There is no attempt to detail the authority of papal or conciliar statements. Nor do I examine issues generally held to be "personal" or to pertain primarily to small entities, such as the family. All of this will need to be argued elsewhere. However, I take as given that the present endeavor has implications for these other tasks.[2]

The U.S. Catholic bishops' 1983 pastoral letter on war and peace, *The Challenge of Peace: God's Promise and Our Response,* is a particularly good document with which to make a case for plausibility and coherence on three counts, each corresponding to a major section of this article.[3] First of all, the debates surrounding the document include clear examples of the deductive-official model, described in part one. Second, the bishops' letter itself is reasonably plausible and coherent. This enables a combination of descriptive commentary on the letter and constructive formulation of the responsive-magisterial approach in part two. Third, the issue of the possession and potential use of nuclear weapons is one requiring the utmost attentiveness and responsiveness of institutions bearing any sort of public responsibility. That the responsive-magisterial approach facilitates this more than the deductive-official alternative is the burden of part three.[4]

The Deductive-Official Model

In the January following the second draft of what was to become *The Challenge of Peace,* representatives of the European bishops' conferences, together with Vatican officials, most notably Cardinal Ratzinger of the Sacred Congregation for the Doctrine of the Faith and Cardinal Casaroli, the Vatican secretary of state, invited representatives of the U.S. bishops' conference to a consultation on the letter. No verbatim text of the meetings was drawn up, but a Vatican-approved synthesis of the exchanges was soon published.[5] Most of the European bishops' interest focuses on the question of whether the documents of bishops' conferences should address the specifics of social issues. The degree and the character of the concern over specifics evidence a deductive-official interpretation of the reason and authority of social documents.

The deductive-official model can be briefly summarized. In a strict deductive understanding of reason, revealed theological truths or doctrines and self-evident philosophical first principles are directly translatable each into the other. The principles are then "applied" to specific situations. Variations include the presence of intermediate principles which link first principles to problem-situations. Still, the criterion is logical entailment. In cases where there is a plurality of legitimate applications, documents should not reason to specifics because they cannot do so with strict logical consistency and therefore with certainty. Not without some tension in the model itself, the deductive form of reasoning is linked to an understanding of authority as the power resting in an individual or group by virtue of their possession of a particular office. Persons in such offices make "pronouncements" on issues of faith (theological truths and doctrines) and set forth "propositions" on matters of morals (universal principles). These pronouncements and propositions are taken to be true because they are uttered by particular persons at certain times and under certain circumstances. Magisterial authority is tightly wedded to juridical function. I will address in detail the tensions within the deductive-official model in part three of this article.

The claim of those who work out of the deductive-official model is that judgments on specifics when there is less than logical entailment involve certain negative effects with regard to forming the consciences of the faithful and shaping the public debate. With the former, specific determinations confuse the faithful on the status of such judgments, implying to the average layperson that the statements carry more authority than they in fact do. This leads to an individualism among the faithful, where persons pick and choose from the teachings that suit them. With the latter, the shaping of the public debate, when the church makes judgments on policy particulars, it loses its uniqueness and becomes merely one institution among others. In so doing, it also loses its influence on other public institutions. I shall assess in detail these effects of specifiic judgments in part three of this article.

The text of the synthesis of the January meeting indicates that the European bishops and Vatican officials closely follow the deductive-official model of reason and authority. Foremost among their concerns is the issue of specifics: "All through the exchange among the participants, a major question kept returning that was formulated in different ways: Should bishops' conferences limit their task to stating general principles or should they also apply these principles to concrete situations, strategies and policies and therefore propose certain practical choices as morally binding?" Resting behind this emphasis on the problem of specifics is a deductive understanding of reason. One begins with revealed doctrine and self-evident principles and only then proceeds, unidirectionally, toward particulars. The European bishops are therefore able to claim, "Substantial consensus must be based on doctrine and does not flow from debate." Assumed is that the church arrives at its doctrine without preceding debate or discussion. The first principles of morality are likewise taken as given. This enables Cardinal Casaroli to argue that one can "deal with true principles of the *moral order* without getting into questions of a technical, political, or any other nature." The result is a sharp distinction, and even separation, between moral principles and their use in particular problem areas. The principles are first independently discerned and *then* "applied" to the situation at hand.[6]

The European bishops link this deductive understanding of reason to a heavily juridical interpretation of authority. Their attention to doctrine and first principles is also a concern about the scope of the rule of their office: "When the bishops propose the doctrine of the church, the faithful are bound in conscience to assent." In referring to the statements of bishops' conferences, Cardinal Casaroli argues, "One must deal with principles that are *certain,* that are *surely and seriously binding* on the Christian and human conscience." The emphasis on the obligation of the faithful to assent to the bishops' propositions implies that to dissent is to necessarily set oneself against the hierarchy. Such an adversarial understanding of plurality again evidences a juridical interpretation of authority. This is once more indicated in the European bishops' insistence that to make judgments on the particulars of a situation is to "take sides."[7]

For the European bishops, the fundamental problem with taking sides on specific issues is that it involves "contingent judgment" rather than the rational certainty and unquestionable authority of doctrines and first principles. Making such judgments has definite negative effects. It confuses the faithful and threatens the unique role of the bishops. Consequently, the bishops' authority is "lessened" and their teaching "obscured or reduced to one element among several in a free debate." The final result is that the influence of the church in society is "weakened."[8]

Both the deductive understanding of reason and the association of authority with the juridical power of particular offices find expression in recent literature. John Finnis's work especially exemplifies the former. In a paper delivered at a conference on Joseph Bernardin's "consistent ethic of life," Finnis seeks to offer a "helpful clarification" of those of the cardinal's formulations which can be "misunderstood."[9] His approach involves four levels, starting with the Christian ethic's central tenet: love of neighbor. "Christian morality's primary principle is 'Love your neighbor as yourself' (understood within the frame of 'Love God above all things' and 'Seek first the Kingdom')."[10] Remaining on this first level, Finnis translates the doctrine into a philosophical principle:

> Philosophically, that first principle of morality can be formulated more abstrusely: One ought to choose and otherwise will those and only those possibilities whose willing is *compatible with integral human fulfillment*, i.e. with the good of all persons and communities, conceived not as a goal attainable by some world-wide billion-year plan but as a guiding ideal which inspires and rectifies practical thinking by the general principles and more specific norms it implies.[11]

Finnis is careful to avoid the trap of "consequentialism" in his understanding of human fulfillment, a matter I shall address in the second part of this article. The point here is that he holds there to be an equivalence and direct translatability between the doctrinal "love of neighbor" and his philosophical principle on the first level of his analysis. The first moral principle has "both its biblical and its more philosophical articulations."[12]

One must, however, proceed beyond this level. "Love of neighbor needs to get down to cases." The second and third levels consist of further specifications of the first principle. The move from love of neighbor to "intermediate" principles such as the Golden Rule is direct and immediate. The relation between the two is "intuitively obvious." The second-level or intermediate principles are then further specified on the third level as "general norms of morality," including "equality before the law" and "no intentional killing of innocents."[13] Finnis offers a succinct summary of his argument from first principle to the norm of no intentional killing of innocents:

> Given the Christian understanding of the significance of choice and action, the traditional norm thus follows from the first principle of Christian ethics: love of neighbor. For human life is intrinsic, not extrinsic, to the human person. A choice against human life is thus a choice against the person: anti-life, therefore anti-person. It is thus incompatible with love of the person, i.e. with the first principle of Christian and rational ethics.
>
> The link I am tracing between the first principle and the specific norm against killing is—like the Golden Rule—an intermediate principle of wider application: One may never choose to destroy any *basic* human good—any intrinsic aspect of *personal* well-being—for the sake of any ulterior good, however important. "Evil" (destruction or damaging of a basic human good) "may not be done" (willed, intended, chosen as means) "for the sake of good."[14]

Finnis's argument is deductive because all intermediate principles and their derived general moral norms are merely specifications of the first moral principle. The crucial move is that from the third level, the general norms of common morality, to specific moral, legal, and political judgments on the fourth and final level. Consistent with the deductive understanding of reason, Finnis views this as a matter of the application of the norms *to* the problem-situations. There are two possibilities here. The first involves cases which yield moral absolutes, such as the prohibitions against abortion and infanticide. In these instances, the movement from general norm to specific prescription is itself logically entailed. No plurality of opinion is morally legitimate. When such is the case, moral dictates on this fourth level directly translate into law:

> Throughout the civilized world, now as in Aquinas' day, the criminal law of homicide closely follows, "translates," indeed transcribes the community's common morality. Each community tries to identify what forms of killing and of death-dealing behavior or omission are *morally* wrongful, and then declares those forms of conduct unlawful or criminal. . . . This virtual coincidence of moral law and state/ national law in relation to the definition and prohibition of homicides (including infanticide) is to be expected and supported.

Thus my question about the social policy that Catholics should support in relation to infanticide has a single, straightforward answer. More generally, the moral absolutes of the tradition have a number of direct "translations" into social policies which in the strictest sense *apply*—are deducible from—the absolute moral norm.[15]

In other cases, the movement from norm to policy is not one of logical entailment. This occurs when the norm is not absolute but instead involves "grave affirmative responsibilities." The obligation to feed the hungry is the primary example. Such requirements allow for a variety of policy responses. Finnis, like the European bishops and Vatican officials, argues that there are "some notable bad side-effects" when bishops address policy particulars in situations involving not moral absolutes, but only affirmative responsibilities. In doing so, he evidences not only the deductive model of reasoning but also the view of authority as "official," demonstrating once again the linkage of methodology and ecclesiology. He too argues that prudential judgments by episcopal bodies confuse the faithful. But the strongest indication of his understanding of authority as associated with particular offices is his argument that bishops cannot make "truly prudential judgments." Only those in political offices can do so. In an extended footnote, he concludes a critical assessment of *The Challenge of Peace* with the comment, "These are all the mistakes of *outsiders*. Truly prudential judgments are the judgments of insiders."[16] Bishops should not address policy particulars because this trespasses on the authority of the *political* officeholders. I shall take up this point again in part three.

The distinction between moral absolutes and grave affirmative responsibilities is crucial when Finnis joins with Joseph Boyle, Jr., and Germain Grisez to assess the morality of deterrence in *Nuclear Deterrence, Morality, and Realism*. Their argument is virtually identical to the one Finnis offers in the consistent-ethic-of-life article. Revealed theological and self-evident philosophical principles entail intermediate principles and, in some instances, specific moral norms. This is the case with deterrence. It comes under the same strict prohibition as infanticide. This is because the movement from intermediate principles to the specific moral norm involves "a deduction which can be formulated in a categorical syllogism." Deterrence threatens to intentionally take the lives of innocent persons. Finnis, Boyle, and Grisez hold that an immoral threat comes under the same judgment as the act it proposes to carry out. Deterrence, therefore, is immoral. For these authors, this condemnation requires immediate unilateral disarmament.[17] They recognize other duties, such as the defense of democratic freedoms, but these are only affirmative responsibilities. The prohibition against killing the innocent is absolute and therefore overriding. When norms conflict, the obligation is clear: avoid intrinsic or absolute moral evils.

> The reality here is twofold: the menace of Soviet power if it were un-deterred by a deterrent system such as actually exists; and the threat to kill the innocent, with its underlying intent, and its guilt. The real-ity, in both respects, is horrible. Every reasonable person wishes to es-cape it. But the only thing one can escape is the guilt. And one can do that only by ceasing to participate in, defend, support, or approve the nuclear deterrent system.[18]

I shall address this avoid-evil/escape-guilt understanding of the moral life more fully in part two. The aim here is to point up how Finnis, Boyle, and Grisez assess deterrence in terms of their moral system. The implications for the ecclesiological question are interesting. Bishops' con-ferences would be allowed to speak to the particulars of the deterrence question *only* if they hold that their conclusion is logically entailed from an absolute principle and if they then proceed to judge the policy nega-tively. In other words, according to this account, church officials must adopt both the method and substantive conclusion of Finnis, Boyle, and Grisez if they are to speak to the problem of deterrence without negative side effects.

One more point is worth noting about the deterrence argument. Be-cause of the absolute status of the principle of not killing the innocent, no matter how infinitesimal the chances of a nuclear exchange and how cer-tain the horrors of life under Soviet domination, the moral judgment against deterrence, and all that this implies for policy, remains the same. Otherwise, the consideration of consequences, rather than the rule of the absolute principle, determines moral choice. If the fundamental norms of Christian ethics are absolute and derivable from self-evident moral prin-ciples, then no shift in our circumstances, however drastic, can lead to a reformulation or a revision of those norms. Finnis is clear on this in his paper. In a section titled "Developing the Tradition Consistently," he argues that any legitimate development of the tradition is not due to the revision or creation of norms in new situations. Rather, it is "an iden-tification, ever more adequate, of *truths* about the human good and human action—about the *intrinsic* demands of love or respect for persons. So I would say that the tradition is developing by penetrating ever more deeply to the full implications of its underlying principles and presuppositions—those I have here been seeking to indicate."[19] As with Cardinal Casaroli and the European bishops, Finnis clearly separates immutable universal principles and their application to the ever-shifting problems of contingent reality. Any alteration in the principles is merely additional "helpful clarification."

The Responsive-Magisterial Approach

The aim in this section is to use the U.S. Catholic bishops' letter, *The Challenge of Peace,* to help set out a viable alternative to the deductive-official model. The responsive-magisterial approach is relatively new, and even the bishops' document is not a pure type. Still, the letter may represent a shift in direction toward a different understanding of reason and authority. Whether it is truly a transitional document is a question for the future to decide. For our purposes it is enough that it is a sufficient example of the present approach to combine descriptive commentary on its structure and content with critical construction of the responsive-magisterial option. Once again, methodology and ecclesiology are linked. The rational activity of response joins with the organizational activity of learning and teaching plausible and coherent responses.

The Rational Activity of Response

The difference between the deductive model and the approach here under consideration is fundamental. In the present case, reason or rationality is not a characteristic of logical systems—deductive or otherwise—but rather of human activity as a whole. And human activity is responsive. Whatever principles, chains of reasoning, or systems of thought a tradition formulates, these are understood to be attempts by the community to respond to the world it finds itself in. The aim of this subsection is to detail, in three stages, what this understanding of rationality involves. First, I will compare *The Challenge of Peace* with H. Richard Niebuhr's *The Responsible Self* in order to descriptively illumine the structure and content of the bishops' letter. Second, I will move in a constructive direction by reconstruing Niebuhr's criteria for adequate response in terms of plausibility and coherence. Third, I will meet anticipated objections to the reconstituted criteria as a way of elaborating possible philosophical underpinnings of the response approach.

THE BISHOPS AND H. RICHARD NIEBUHR

One of the most notable aspects of *The Challenge of Peace* is that its overarching language is that of "promise," or "challenge," and "response." This is first of all evident in the subtitle of the document, "God's Promise and Our Response." The bishops make clear their intended meaning: "Peace and war must always be seen in light of God's intervention in human affairs and our response to that intervention. Both are elements within the ongoing revelation of God's will for creation."[20] God's intervention is at once promise and challenge, and our fundamental obligation is to respond accordingly. The bishops therefore set up the framework of the document by interpreting the nature of responsiveness in general biblical terms in the first major section and by calling persons in their particular vocations to respond in the last section. Together, these form an *inclusio* around the moral reasoning about nuclear armaments and policy choices which constitute the middle parts of the letter.

The moral language of response, responsiveness, and responsibility is relatively new. The term *responsibility* emerged in philosophical circles in the debates on freedom and necessity in the nineteenth century. It then developed to address issues of both the attribution and appropriation of moral obligation. Twentieth-century theological ethics has broadened the concept to range over the entirety of the moral life as its fundamental norm.[21] It has subsumed the narrower understanding of responsibility under a more inclusive interpretation which characterizes all of reality in terms of response or responsiveness. Here, the works of Martin Buber, Dietrich Bonhoeffer, Bernard Häring, Robert Johann, and H. Richard Niebuhr are foremost in importance.[22] Though comparing the bishops with any of these authors would be helpful, interpreting the document in terms of Niebuhr's thought is most illuminative of its structure and content.

In the prologue to his work, Niebuhr boldly states his fundamental descriptive premise: "All life has the character of responsiveness, I maintain." The rest of the book details just what this implies for the moral agent. Most importantly, it involves a change in the basic question of the moral life from those posed by deontological and teleological approaches.

Rather than ask, "What is my goal, ideal or telos?" or "What is the law and what is the first law of my life?" (as in the deductive model), an ethics of response begins with the query, "What is going on?" Niebuhr here often invokes the same language of challenge and response found in the bishops' letter. He writes, "We try to understand history less by asking about the ideals toward which societies and their leaders directed their efforts or about the laws they were obeying and more by inquiring into the challenges in their natural and social environment to which the societies were responding."[23]

Niebuhr elaborates four basic elements of this challenge/response morphology of the moral life. The *response* itself to the actions upon us is the first element. Second is the fact of our *interpretation* of those actions. Niebuhr calls the third element *accountability,* our taking into consideration that our responses prompt further responses from others. Our response is always "made in anticipation of reply." Fourth and finally is *social solidarity*. Action is responsible when it is response "in a continuing discourse or interaction among beings forming a continuing society." At this point Niebuhr emphasizes what we have been highlighting about the responsive approach: our aim is not the immutability of our principles but rather the continuity of the traditions of which we are a member and with which we interact as we seek to respond to what is going on. Responsibility "implies continuity in the community of agents to which response is being made." Niebuhr calls action which responds in accordance with all of these elements of responsibility a "fitting" response.[24]

One interpretation of *The Responsible Self* is that it is a phenomenological analysis of the moral life.[25] Yet Niebuhr's description also has a normative aspect: "Responsibility affirms: 'God is acting in all actions upon you. So respond to all actions upon you as to respond to his action.' " Thus when he depicts the fitting action as "the one that fits into a total interaction as response and as interpretation of further response" and writes that such action "is alone conducive to the good and alone is right," he not only describes but also, on a general level, prescribes.[26] Fittingness of response, rather than logical entailment from first principles, is the fundamental criterion of the moral life.[27]

There is more that one could detail of Niebuhr's concept of responsibility, but the above is enough to argue for a significant congruity between Niebuhr and the bishops in both structure and content. The opening paragraphs of *The Challenge of Peace* indicate that the bishops, like

Niebuhr, begin with the attempt to address the question, What is going on? Quoting the Second Vatican Council, they initiate their document with a description of a world with nuclear weapons:

> "The whole human race faces a moment of supreme crisis in its advance toward maturity." Thus the Second Vatican Council opened its treatment of modern warfare. Since the council, the dynamic of the nuclear arms race has intensified. . . .
>
> As bishops and pastors ministering in one of the major nuclear nations, we have encountered this terror in the minds and hearts of our people—indeed, we share it. . . .
>
> The crisis of which we speak arises from this fact: nuclear war threatens the existence of our planet; this is a more menacing threat than any the world has known.[28]

The nuclear situation itself then prompts the bishops to adopt a *response* approach. This is clear if we note that Niebuhr argues that the practical life experiences of social emergencies and personal suffering necessitate the responsibility approach to ethics. Again, the challenge/response language is in evidence in Niebuhr: "The emergence of modern America out of the Civil War when measures were adopted in response to challenges that the founding fathers had not foreseen . . . such events give evidence in the social sphere of the extent to which active, practical self-definition issues from response to challenge rather than from the pursuit of an ideal or from adherence to some ultimate laws."[29] Teleological and deontological approaches do not adequately address emergency and suffering because such situations have significant aspects not currently under our control and obey laws different from our own.

The bishops' language of crisis in the opening paragraphs expresses their concern that the situation is indeed an emergency. Their reference to "this terror in the minds and hearts of our people" recognizes intense suffering. Throughout the pastoral letter, they emphasize that the destructive capacity of nuclear weapons presents us with a situation unique in history.[30] They do not abandon the tradition—its modes of reasoning, deontological or teleological; its systems of thought, just war and pacifist; its fundamental principles, noncombatant immunity and proportionality—but they understand clearly that traditional modes of reasoning, systems of thought, and principles must be subsumed under the practical necessity and the moral obligation to respond to the challenge at hand.

Following their initial description of what is going on and their turn to a response approach, the bishops draw from their tradition to give a biblical-theological *interpretation* in the first major section of the document.[31] They use a theological mode of discourse to offer the most inclusive possible construal of the situation. Here again they closely follow Niebuhr's ethics. He argues in *The Responsible Self* that the crucial contribution of religious communities to public discussion of social issues is their overarching interpretation of what is going on: "The great religions in general, and Christianity in particular . . . make their impact on us by calling into question our whole conception of what is fitting—that is, of what really fits in—by questioning our picture of the context into which we now fit our actions."[32] The bishops view their contribution in just this way: "In the face of this frightening and highly speculative debate on a matter involving millions of human lives, we believe the most effective contribution or moral judgment is to introduce perspectives by which we can assess the empirical debate."[33]

The perspective within which the bishops interpret the debate is a biblical one. It is here that the language of promise and response, gift and call, articulated in the scriptural terms of covenantal fidelity, is most prevalent. Notable is the bishops' insistence that the theological language is not directly translatable into other modes of discourse, philosophical or otherwise. In reference to "certain key moral principles," the bishops state, "These norms do not exhaust the gospel vision."[34] The metaphors of *vision* and *image* dominate the theological discourse, indicating that such language does not provide us with principles, but rather construes or interprets the context within which our use of principles will be appropriate.[35] The bishops stay with visual metaphors, primarily the phrase *in light of,* when they relate the theological to the other modes of discourse. Once again, "Peace and war must always be seen in light of God's intervention in human affairs and our response to that intervention."[36] The use of this language recalls a document, commissioned by the Federal Council of Churches, which Niebuhr had a major hand in writing, "The Relation of the Church to the War in Light of the Christian Faith."[37] For the bishops, the biblical vision, in light of which we are to act, does not translate directly into philosophical principles but rather interprets—or better, illumines—a context which then provides "an urgent direction" for our response.[38]

If we are to take this formulation of the role of theological discourse in the bishops' letter seriously, then we must understand the other modes of discourse—philosophical/ethical and political—not to provide, insofar as possible, a chain of deduction from self-evident truths to policy choices, but rather to function heuristically to help clarify what constitutes a fitting response to particular problem-situations. Recall that the theological discourse at the beginning of the document interprets what is going on in the broadest possible promise/response context and that the pastoral discourse at the end calls for specific responses. Together they form the *inclusio*. The purpose of the intervening modes of discourse is therefore to join interpreted promise and challenge to called response. I shall elaborate on this point in the next subsection.

The bishops' letter exhibits not only Niebuhr's concepts of what is going on, response, and interpretation, but also that of *accountability*, the recognition that one's response is always in anticipation of the responses of others. Indeed, the bishops not only anticipate but repeatedly make explicit that they seek to catalyze such responses: "This letter is therefore both an invitation and a challenge to Catholics in the United States to join with others in shaping the conscious choices and deliberate policies required in this 'moment of crisis.' " They state the desire that their document be "a first step" and "a starting point and inspiration." They further realize that this requires much of themselves: "We are prepared and eager to participate in our country in the ongoing public debate on moral grounds." Ultimately, they articulate their commitment to accountability in terms of their faith: "To be disciples of Jesus requires that we continually go beyond where we now are."[39]

Finally, the bishops aim to make their document a living example of *social solidarity*, the fact that responsible action is, again in Niebuhr's terms, "interaction among beings forming a continuing society." They do so in two ways. First, they seek to interact with others in present society: "Building peace within and among nations is the work of many individuals and institutions; it is the fruit of ideas and decisions taken in the political, cultural, economic, social, military, and legal sectors of life." This point is repeated frequently throughout the letter.[40] While other documents of the Catholic tradition may have made similar declarations, the two-year consultative process by which the bishops sought advice from persons of all sectors of society makes the present letter a genuine example of social solidarity.[41] The difference is that although documents since Pius XII have explicitly spoken *to* the wider public or set of publics, the bishops here situate themselves *among* these publics. Even commentators who strongly disagree with the contents of the letter have commended the open process.[42] Second, the bishops also exhibit solidarity when they appropriate the accumulated wisdom of their tradition in their effort to respond to the situation at hand. In this way, they demonstrate their membership in a continuing society of persons. The bishops consider themselves to have "both the obligation and the opportunity to share and interpret the moral and religious wisdom of the Catholic tradition."[43] They fulfill their role by drawing upon teachings concerning the theological context of peace, the political order, and the use of force, particularly as these are set forth in the Second Vatican Council's *Pastoral Constitution on the Church in the Modern World*.[44] (Significantly, the *Pastoral Constitution* has been called "the great charter of the ethic of responsibility.")[45] This accumulated wisdom is the source of the continuity in the community's rational activity of response over time to changing problem-situations. Niebuhr makes the point aptly:

> Not with timeless laws of never-changing nature or of a pure human, unhistorical reason, does the self come to its present encounters. It comes rather with images and patterns of interpretation, with attitudes of trust and suspicion, accumulated in its historical past. . . . The remembered images are the product not, in the first place, of its own past encounters but of a society which has taught it a language with names and explicit or implicit metaphors and with an implicit logic.[46]

The effort to conserve such an accumulated tradition stands in contrast to the deductive-official attempt to isolate immutable principles.

The above comparison between Niebuhr and the bishops is sufficient, I believe, to descriptively illumine the response approach of the pastoral letter. I take it to be now evident that the similarities are in fact often striking. My task now is to draw upon these observations while moving in a more constructive direction. The criterion of fittingness needs to be further developed in terms faithful to *The Responsible Self* and *The Challenge of Peace*.

FROM FITTINGNESS TO PLAUSIBILITY AND COHERENCE

The aim of this subsection is to reconstitute the criterion of fittingness in a way that renders more explicit several crucial aspects of the ethics of responsibility. I do so using the terms *plausibility* and *coherence*.

Plausibility emphasizes the fact that human action is a social response, and is therefore to be validated publicly. What one finds to be fitting must be presented in public in a way that is plausible. I shall detail what philosophical commitments are involved in plausibility in the next subsection. For now it is enough to point out that Niebuhr articulates this fact of the publicness of responsibility through his elaboration of accountability and social solidarity. In accordance with these elements of responsibility, the bishops situate themselves in the wisdom of their tradition and from there engage persons in other sectors of life. Human action arises out of a social matrix and anticipates further public response.

Plausibility also makes it explicit that all moral methodologies (deontological and teleological), principles (e.g., no intentional killing of innocents), and the systems of thought which they constitute (the varieties of just-war theories and pacifism) are subsumed under the rubric of responsibility, the rational action of response. All are brought under the activity of the community, the living tradition, as it seeks to respond to what is going on. This does not eliminate distinctive methods, principles, and systems, but it does mean a quite different understanding of their genesis and value than that offered by the deductive model. On the present understanding, they are introduced by communities at various times to aid in the response to particular problem-situations. Their enduring value depends on their ability to continue to serve in this way.

More specifically, the function of methods, principles, and systems is a heuristic one. Their role is illuminative and connective. They serve to illumine or highlight plausible responses and to connect to those responses an interpretation of what is going on. This is as opposed to their prescriptive and justificatory function in a deductive model. In this latter approach, they, of their own accord, prescribe and therefore justify a particular act. Reason is a matter of applying the deductive method to all cases. The response approach instead emphasizes that the major part of rationality is in recognizing which combination of methods, principles, and systems is called for by a particular problem-situation. Deductive argumentation is just one option in this understanding of reasoning. It has value insofar as it helps illumine and connect.[47] However, use of an exclusively deductive mode of reasoning is irrational in situations which have so significantly changed from that of the model's original use as to render the approach obscurant and fragmental rather than illuminative and connective. I will provide more on this point in part three.

The response approach to reason has specific implications for present debates around the status of modes of reasoning, principles, and systems.

With the first of these, the understanding of rationality as a dimension of the activity or practice of a community relativizes the debate between "proportionalists" and their detractors. The debate is indeed important. However, the issue is not which method is "better" in some absolute sense but rather which one, or even which combination of the two, best functions to illumine our responses and connect them to our interpretation of what is going on. When Niebuhr sets the responsibility approach over against the teleological "man-the-maker" and deontological "man-the-citizen" alternatives, his primary criticism is not that the other options are unreasonable per se, but that either one taken alone offers an incomplete description of the moral life. Once this point is understood, then one can incorporate both teleology and deontology into a responsibility approach.[48]

The just-war tradition, for example, combines both goal-oriented and rule-oriented judgments. This is clearly evident in the bishops' letter. Their condemnation of counterpopulation warfare is the result of a deontological application of the principle of noncombatant immunity: "No Christian can rightfully carry out orders or policies deliberately aimed at killing non-combatants. We make this judgment at the beginning of our treatment of nuclear strategy because the defense of the principle of noncombatant immunity is so important for the ethic of war and because the nuclear age has posed such extreme problems for the principle." The bishops' treatment of the initiation of nuclear war and limited nuclear war, however, involves teleological considerations of proportionality and reasonable hope of success: "Former public officials have testified that it is improbable that any nuclear war could actually be kept limited."[49] The claim of an ethic of response is that the elimination of either one of these types of judgments would impoverish the tradition. Allowing for both avoids the excesses in strategic thought when a strict deontological model tends toward immediate unilateral disarmament and when an exclusively teleological approach leads to indiscriminately targeting population centers.

When one views *principles* and *systems of thought* as instances of the rational activity of a community, one sets them within the overall context of their development in the tradition of which they are a part. It is then more accurate to refer to, say, just-war theories in the plural or the just-war tradition than to a singular theory.[50] The principles of the tradition are the result of the crystallization of the community's accumulated wisdom at particular times. The fundamental just-war question is not then "How do we apply these principles?" but rather "Given our present resources and the problem-situation confronting us, how must we order society and limit the use of force so that we can most fully respond to God's promise and challenge of peace?" Again, the bishops insist, "Peace and war must always be seen in light of God's intervention in human affairs and our response to that intervention."[51] This understanding of the just-war tradition includes the possibility that the present resources may be found wanting and in need of revision or development. This point is more fully addressed in my discussion of coherence.

Coherence is a function of plausibility. The plausible response is one in which an interpretation of what is going on is linked to the rational action of the community. The truth value of the methods, principles, and systems of thought is in whether they *coherently* join promise and challenge to response. An incoherent response will not likely be plausible. As with the criterion of plausibility, I will detail the philosophical commitments of coherence in the next subsection. The aim here is to use the concept to make explicit certain elements of the responsibility approach in the bishops' letter and Niebuhr's thought. These elements include the use of multiple modes of discourse and the possibility of the revision and development of the methods, principles, and systems of thought mentioned above.

Rather than directly translating theological doctrine into philosophical first principles and working through the problem of war as a matter of deduction, the bishops use multiple modes of discourse, each with a different relation to the others, to aid in discerning plausible responses: "The Catholic social tradition, as exemplified in the *Pastoral Constitution* and recent papal teachings, is a mix of biblical, theological, and philosophical elements which are brought to bear upon the concrete problems of the day."[52] The document is structured so that one or the other of these modes of discourse predominates in each of the sections, opening with the theological and then moving through the philosophical/ethical and the political to the pastoral. Again, the theological discourse interprets the ultimate context within which persons of different vocations, addressed in the closing pastoral section, are to respond. The bishops use visual metaphors ("in light of") instead of reducing the theological to the philosophical, while still maintaining the influence of the former ("provides an urgent direction") on the latter. The philosophical/ethical and political modes of discourse then serve to connect biblically articulated covenanted promise to pastoral response.[53] They help to specify which responses might be plausible. As the adherents of the deductive model recognize, logical entailment from ethical principles to political choices is not always, or even frequently, possible. The point to be made from the response perspective is that this fact does not count against specific political judgments being made in church documents. All of the modes of discourse are subject, in varying degrees, to significant changes in what is going on (such as the development of nuclear weapons) and therefore to the need for revision and development. Thus our second point under the heading of coherence.

The claim of the deductive model is that the universal self-evident principles and the intermediate principles derivable from them are fundamentally immune from the contingencies of human life. Again, for Cardinal Casaroli, one can "deal with true principles of the moral order without getting into questions of a technical, political, or any other nature." Finnis asserts that any change in the tradition is due to "penetration ever more deeply to the full implications of its underlying principles and presuppositions." The principles themselves are immutable, subject only to clarification. Not even drawing comment is the possibility of revising theological doctrine or moral methodologies, a foreclosed prospect.

The responsibility approach offers a different account. Because our actions are in response to specific circumstances, significant shifts in those circumstances have an impact not only on our formulations of plausible and coherent options but also on the responses themselves. Alterations in our articulations then follow upon changes in our response. Moreover, since what is going on influences the entirety of our response, no mode of discourse is in principle exempt from the possibility of revision. All of this is implied by Niebuhr's understanding of accountability.[54]

The bishops describe the presence and possible use of nuclear weapons as a situation which is qualitatively new in political and military history. They quote the Second Vatican Council in recognizing that this set of circumstances calls for "a completely fresh reappraisal of war." This requires not an abandonment but a thorough reassessment of previous teachings: "The task before us is not simply to repeat what we have said before; it is first to consider anew whether and how our religious-moral tradition can assess, direct, contain, and, we hope, help to eliminate the threat posed to the human family by the nuclear arsenals of the world."[55] The point here is that the tradition, as inherited from previous responses to the problem of war, is not fully adequate to address what is now going on.

The bishops' reconsideration of the tradition is perhaps most thorough with the theological mode of discourse. Absent are any claims that consensus flows from doctrine and not debate. In its place is a recognition that the present theological task necessitates exchange: "We address theologians in a particular way, because we know that we have only begun the journey toward a theology of peace; without your specific contributions this desperately needed dimension of our faith will not be realized. Through your help we may provide new vision and wisdom for church and state."[56] The just-war tradition, once set within a theological understanding of peace, has lost its bearings due to the rise of autonomous nation-states. Now, with the development of the nascent stages of international interdependence and the capacity for indiscriminate nuclear destruction, a retrieval and renewal of the theological context is at once both possible and necessary.[57]

In the philosophical/ethical mode of discourse, significant changes in circumstance affect methodologies, principles, and systems of thought. I shall this time address these in reverse order. The most significant development in terms of *systems of thought* is the increased openness to the pacifist option for individuals as an alternative to the just-war tradition. As late as 1956, Pius XII rejected conscientious objection, basing his argument on the country's duty to defend itself.[58] The Second Vatican Council's *Pastoral Constitution* and the U.S. Catholic bishops' 1968 document *Human Life in Our Day* reversed this foreclosure on pacifism, while still affirming the nation-state's duty of self-defense.[59] *The Challenge of Peace* reaffirms this latter position, particularly the point that political bodies as a whole are still obliged to defend themselves. But it also goes a step further by arguing that the tradition, in responding to the problem of the possession and use of nuclear weapons, needs to understand the just-war and pacifist alternatives as "complementary" and "distinct but interdependent." Their argument is, to use the terms of this article, that both traditions are necessary in order to fully illumine the community's response: "We believe the two perspectives support and complement one another, each preserving the other from distortion." The bishops give theological warrant for this position by arguing that the tension between God's kingdom and human history generates complexity in the tradition, creating a situation in which a certain diversity of options is not only legitimate but desirable.[60] David Hollenbach, Francis X. Meehan, and Duane K. Friesen have all argued that this understanding of just war and pacifism constitutes a genuine development of the tradition.[61]

Shifts in circumstances can affect received *principles* in a number of ways, sometimes involving only their being temporarily overridden, as with the presumption against war that the bishops hold to be at the center of just-war teaching.[62] The presumption has the status of a prima facie duty. In other instances, older principles are simply reinterpreted for new circumstances. This is the case when the bishops relate the criteria of competent authority to democratic governments and modern revolution, last resort to the present need for a stronger United Nations, and both noncombatant immunity and proportionality to the problem of the destructive capacity of nuclear weapons. Elsewhere, situational changes prompt a retrieval of norms which have been neglected in modern versions of just-war thought. The growth of interdependence between nation-states and the consequent relativization of individual claims of sovereignty make possible the bishops' renewal of the principle of comparative justice. Most significantly, unforeseen circumstances may necessitate the creation of new principles, such as those the bishops devise to set the limits on their "strictly conditioned moral acceptance of deterrence."[63] David Hollenbach has given the clearest statement of these principles: "First, any new policy proposal must make nuclear war less likely than the policies presently in effect rather than more likely. Second, any new policy proposal must increase the possibility of arms reduction rather than decrease this possibility."[64]

The immediate implication of the influence of circumstances on principles is that the strict separation of universal principles and contingent applications is relativized. The most one could expect is for the patterns of problem-situations and communal responses to have sufficient continuity over time and between traditions to be considered, for practical purposes, universal. When such is the case, a straightforward application of previously formed principles may be all that is necessary. It is possible in limited situations for a deductive approach to be sufficiently illuminative and connective. But even here, the principles are always subject to changing circumstances, and therefore to revision. Thus, there is a distinction between principles and their use in specific problem areas, but it is a relationship where the two parts are always interactive.

It is at this point that the bishops' letter shows some tensions. In one brief subsection in particular, the language of "universal principles" and their "application" is quite strong.[65] Two comments are in order. First, this language was considerably hardened in the drafts after the meeting with the European bishops and Vatican officials. In other words, it was a response to the January meeting and in anticipation of further responses from the same interlocutors. The hardening of the language was itself an effort to exhibit social solidarity and accountability. Second, if the distinction between principles and their use in specific circumstances is taken as absolute, then, as indicated above, for the most part the bishops do not follow it in practice. To the degree that they accept a strict separation of principle and situation as their self-understanding of their method, they reason better than they know.[66]

Still, there is one principle that the bishops do specifically insist is absolute—no direct killing of innocents: "The lives of innocent persons may never be taken directly, regardless of the purpose alleged for doing so." This insistence has immediate implications for *methodology* because this particular principle has been historically articulated within a particular ethical framework, that of deductivism. In the bishops' case, the *imago Dei* theological doctrine translates into the philosophical statement of the dignity of humans, the statement from which one derives the prohibition against directly killing the innocent.[67]

The traditional mechanism through which moralists have avoided revision of this principle is that of double effect. Briefly stated, double effect contends that an act has more than one effect, and that the only effect the agent is morally responsible for is the one he or she directly intends. The rest are, if evil, only regrettable indirect side effects. The debates around what is more exactly meant by *direct* and *indirect* intention are too complex to detail here.[68] The double-effect mechanism itself developed in large part in response to a need within the community to precisely determine an agent's culpability in the sacrament of penance. It has since gained, through time and use, the status of a principle. The point from the response approach is that whatever the original purpose in developing double effect, its use in reasoning about the possession and use of nuclear weapons has cut in two opposite directions, neither of which are satisfactory. On the one hand, double effect has allowed some thinkers to argue that military installations in large population centers may be attacked—even while the absolute prohibition against killing the innocent remains intact—because the deaths of noncombatants are only indirectly intended. This is the case in Paul Ramsey's thought.[69] On the other hand, double effect has been used to argue for immediate unilateral disarmament. Whatever atrocities may occur as a result of capitulation to Soviet power are merely a side effect of avoiding the guilt of the intention to kill the innocent, guilt involved in the policy of deterrence. Finnis, Boyle, and Grisez make this argument. Both positions avoid revising the principle against directly killing the innocent, at the cost of discounting as morally irrelevant large portions of what is going on. My interpretation of the pastoral letter is that the bishops recognize this problem. Therefore, although they use the term *direct,* they do not use the mechanism of double effect.

The problem is that the disuse of double effect puts considerable pressure on the claim of the absolute status of the principle of no direct killing of innocents. There is no way to divert those aspects of the situation which are in tension with the claim. One of the most persistent criticisms of the pastoral letter is that the absolute status of the principle is incoherent with the conditioned moral acceptance of deterrence.[70] To be coherent, the bishops have to acknowledge that the prohibition on the intent to kill noncombatants is theoretically subject to being overridden, reinterpreted, or revised. At the very least, it must function in conjunction with, and not simply override, other principles in conflict situations. The deductive mode of reasoning from the *imago Dei* doctrine to the noncombatant principle is still adequate to the degree that it illumines certain aspects of what is going on: primarily the concern that modern life in general and preparation for potential nuclear warfare in particular work to cheapen the value of the human person. There are therefore good reasons to argue that the prohibition against intentionally killing innocents should perdure. The limits of the principle are in evidence when it begins to obscure, particularly when taken as absolute, important dimensions of the problem-situation.

The latter occurs in the argument of Finnis, Boyle, and Grisez. Again, they recognize that the defense of democratic freedom is a grave affirmative responsibility. But the duty to avoid the intention to kill the innocent is absolute and therefore overriding in any situation in which it is applicable. Where an absolute principle and affirmative responsibilities come into conflict, the former, always stated in the negative, is trump. The upshot is that in such situations, action is ruled by the dictate "Avoid guilt."[71] All other aspects of what is going on are *morally* irrelevant. From the perspective of a responsibility ethic, this construal of conflict situations involves a truncated understanding of the moral life. There is more involved in responding to conflict situations than avoiding evil, and the relevance of a traditionally invoked norm such as the prohibition against the intention to kill innocents for a specific problem-situation does not render all other aspects of the situation morally impertinent. An ethic which above all else seeks to avoid guilt is therefore implausible. When one insists that the loss of civil and political liberties following upon the decision to unilaterally disarm is a mere side effect, a permitted but not committed evil, the tradition is no longer responding to the whole of what is going on. Rather, it has replaced its rational activity of response with the irrational activity of trying to preserve, as absolute, principles and methodologies which arose in response to quite different situations and which now only obscure and fragment rather than illumine and connect.

The implausible response, as we stated before, will also be incoherent. The irony of Finnis, Boyle, and Grisez's insistence on the absolute status of the prohibition against the intention to kill the innocent and the consequent requirement to unilaterally disarm is that it shifts attention away from significant manifestations of the value the principle was originally formed to protect. These authors readily admit that disarmament by the United States would open its citizens to human rights violations on the part of the Soviet bloc.[72] But, they argue, the only pertinent factor for them is NATO's—and therefore our—conditional intention to use nuclear weapons. The problem is that no matter how remote the possibilities of use may be, and regardless of how inevitable Soviet harm to unprotected and innocent citizens of Western nations may become, the absolute principle—functioning in an ethic which in conflict situations seeks above all else to avoid guilt—requires that we unilaterally disarm. When such is the case, the effort to preserve a particular formulation of a principle under the claim of its absolute status undermines important manifestations—in this case that of the lives of innocent American persons—of the reality, the real value, that it was originally meant to preserve.[73]

Whatever the bishops claim for the principle of no direct killing of innocents, their recognition of the implausibility and incoherence of proposals for unilateral disarmament leads them to use the principle in a way that is not absolute as understood by Finnis, Boyle, and Grisez. Rather it functions as it should in a responsibility ethic: to direct us to a value which requires illumination given the tendency of modern warfare to cheapen human worth. The bishops use other principles—for instance, the duty of a nation to defend itself—to bring to light other aspects of what is going on. Responsible activity is possible only when persons and communities construe circumstances as broadly and completely as possible, without discounting crucial dimensions of the situation as morally irrelevant.

Systems of thought, principles, and methodologies are therefore all subject to reconsideration and even revision. This fact leads to a quite different understanding of the development of doctrine than that put forth by the deductive-official model. Reinterpretations and revisions reflect real changes in response, which follow upon shifts in God's challenge in problem-situations. This is clear in the bishops' insistence on the "ongoing revelation of God's will for creation," their recognition that the just-war tradition "has evolved," and their desire to "continue and develop the teaching on peace and war." Throughout the document, their concern is not only with how but also with whether the tradition as inherited is adequate for responding to the problem of nuclear warfare.[74] These statements, taken together with the way the systems of thought, principles, and methodologies in fact function in the document, imply that from the response perspective, the claim that development is simply a clarification of immutable principles is itself, in the technical sense of the term used here, implausible.

Given the development of theological and philosophical/ethical modes of discourse in response to changing problem-situations, the task of the criteria for social documents is not only to assess particular claims but also to aid in the responsible evolution of church teaching. The liability of claims of absolute status for principles is that they inordinately resist alteration in the face of new realities; the community's activity becomes irrational. Change then comes, if at all, only as the result of convulsions in the tradition.[75] The responsibility approach allows change to occur more gradually and self-reflectively.[76] The task now is to constructively set out philosophical underpinnings of plausibility and coherence. In doing so, I aim to show that these criteria facilitate change without falling into the traps of consequentialism or relativism.

PLAUSIBILITY AND COHERENCE: PHILOSOPHICAL CONSIDERATIONS

In this subsection I shall address anticipated objections to plausibility and coherence, as a way of locating the response approach philosophically. The aim is that of construction rather than commentary. My sense is that the bishops, if asked, would most likely affirm a rather straightforward realism, of the sort generally associated with natural law, as their moral epistemology. At the same time, the reasoning of their document is in terms of response. Natural law is referred to only twice, and remains undeveloped.[77] This much is clear: the bishops do not share the neo-scholastic construal of natural law theory as providing a foundation for the immutable principles of a static order. They would, I imagine, want to combine response and natural law, a project Bernard Häring has taken up at length.[78]

But again, my task is constructive. Therefore, I wish to engage a broader range of conversation partners. I shall draw upon two moral philosophers—Morton White and Hilary Putnam—to address the objections.

Objection: Plausibility and coherence entail a form of consequentialism.

Response: Though the term *consequentialism* is primarily used in Roman Catholic moral theology, the issue is one that arises in various forms in Protestant ethics (the "situation ethics" and "norm versus context" debates in the 1960s)[79] and moral philosophy (teleology vs. deontology). The charge is particularly difficult to field in the Roman Catholic discussion because it is often made without precision. Proportionalism, which allows for the consideration of consequences in the assessment of the moral status of an act, is frequently conflated with consequentialism or utilitarianism, where the end result of an act is decisive in determining its status.[80]

Even thinkers as careful as Finnis, Boyle, and Grisez give what under scrutiny appears to be two accounts of consequentialism. The first identifies as consequentialist all moral theories which reject the claim that there are absolute moral norms deducible from self-evident first principles: "Some have suggested that the norm forbidding the intentional killing of non-combatants should not be considered a moral absolute, but only a non-absolute norm, or a convention justified by its utility. Even if those who hold this position do not profess consequentialism, their thesis fits into consequentialist defences of deterrence." Those who do not profess their consequentialism of this sort are "crypto-consequentialists."[81] I shall call this position "non-absolutism," meaning a theory which holds that no singularly formulated norm is free from the possibility of revision. Their second account of consequentialism is a more specific definition: it is a theory which holds that "a correct moral judgment prescribes the choice of that option likely to lead to an overall preferable state of affairs—one in which benefits are maximized and harms minimized." To calculate the maximization of benefits, the consequentialist must hold that all goods are commensurable. At bottom, the theory is a form of cost-benefit analysis.[82] I shall retain the term *consequentialism* for this approach.

I choose different terms for the two accounts because they identify options which are not fully overlapping. More specifically, not every form of non-absolutism constitutes consequentialism. W. D. Ross's understanding of prima facie duties is a case in point. While not absolute in Finnis, Boyle, and Grisez's sense, the norms are still incommensurable, and their use in moral reasoning certainly does not reduce to cost-benefit analysis.[83] If we accept the non-absolutist account alone, then it is clear that a response ethic is included. But the use of the term *consequentialist* is misleading for the very reason just given: far from all non-absolutism fits under the second and more descriptively accurate definition of consequentialism. This second account proves the more interesting charge because it illumines characteristic differences between the response and deductive approaches.

From the perspective of the response approach, the claim that plausibility and coherence involve consequentialism is above all misplaced. The charge still takes the issues of consequentialism vs. deductivism as fundamental rather than heuristic. As stated earlier, the challenge-response morphology and its criteria of plausibility and coherence subsume the concerns of the consequentialist debate. One may use either the consequentialist or the deductive method or both, depending on their heuristic value in connecting the interpretation of the problem-situation to the moral response. Because responses feed back into and sometimes revise methods and principles, a strict absolutist deductivism, which takes its method as well as its basic principles to be immune from revision, is excluded. But what Morton White terms "hypothetical-deductive" arguments can be quite illuminative.

White views the function of argument in a way analogous to the response approach. Principles, methods, and systems of thought are interpretive devices which link sense experience (what is going on) to moral feelings or the moral sense (moral response). The deductive arguments are "hypothetical" because one can have "recalcitrant" moral feelings which prompt the revision of principles, methods, and systems. In situations where no presently available principles apply, concern for consequences can shape one's actions until, in time, new principles are forged.[84] This seems to be the case in the bishops' response to deterrence. It is a new problem-situation, one which the wisdom of the just-war tradition, as it stands, cannot fully address. In their efforts to reconnect sense experience and their collective moral sense, the bishops create the specific guidelines for acceptable deterrence. All along, the moral sense is recalcitrant to the idea of immediate unilateral disarmament, prompting the pursuit of other alternatives.

Given what we have thus far said about the response approach, we would want to modify White's contribution. He places too much exclusive emphasis on moral feelings as the basis of revision and not enough stress on how long-standing moral arguments—the wisdom of the tradition—should shape moral feelings in return. His construal of the moral agent is always as one who is a "normal person under normal circumstances."[85] Therefore, he talks very little about formation. From the response perspective, then, White insufficiently develops the social dimension of responsibility. The communities which constitute the fact of social solidarity for us shape our moral responses.

This much said, White's hypothetical-deductive approach indicates that, in certain cases, deductivism may be sufficiently illuminative. Such instances usually involve relatively stable problem-situations and therefore little need to reconsider principles. The approach also evidences that in circumstances of relatively rapid change, such as that of the continuing development of nuclear weapons technology, a strict deductivism, where the method as well as the principles are held to be absolute, is inadequate. It lacks sufficient flexibility to respond to developing circumstances. In the effort to elevate the status of a particular method and principle, the strict deductive approach conceals both significant dimensions of what is going on and potential resources in the tradition. It is, in a word, unresponsive.

Finnis, Boyle, and Grisez's virtual identification of non-absolutism with consequentialism threatens to obscure the issues which the two terms separately designate. While the charge that the response approach is consequentialist is misplaced, the concern that it is non-absolutist stands firm, and raises a second possible objection that I must address.

Objection: Plausibility and coherence entail a form of relativism.
Response: The fact that the non-absolutism of plausibility and co-

herence allows moral responses to feed back into and revise principles does relativize—while it still retains—the principle/application distinction inherited from the strict deductive model of reasoning. Perdurability and continuity, rather than immutability and universality, are the marks of sound principles. Still, there are constraints on what constitutes a plausible and coherent response. Therefore, a response approach is not an example of radical relativism. It places limits on legitimate plurality while allowing for the rational development of the tradition.

One way to philosophically locate plausibility and coherence is through an epistemological theory that Hilary Putnam calls "internal" or "pragmatic" realism.[86] The basic claim is that the questions "What objects does the world consist of?" and therefore "How shall we respond?" make sense only within a theory or description of the problem-situation— thus the term *internal realism.*[87] This is as opposed to "metaphysical" or "external" realism, where "the world consists of some fixed totality of mind-independent objects. There is exactly one true and complete description of 'the way the world is.' " Putnam calls this the externalist perspective because "its favorite point of view is the God's Eye point of view."[88]

Putnam pushes even further Niebuhr's insistence that the fitting response can be discerned only within a description or interpretation of what is going on. Reality and interpretative schemes are inseparable: "The mind and the world jointly make up the mind and the world."[89] While this allows for plurality, what Putnam calls "conceptual relativity," it does not entail a radical relativism:

> Internal realism is, at bottom, just the insistence that realism is *not* incompatible with conceptual relativity. One can be *both* a realist *and* a conceptual relativist. Realism (with a small "r") . . . takes our familiar commonsense scheme, as well as our scientific and artistic and other schemes, at face value, without helping itself to the notion of the thing "in itself". . . . Conceptual relativity sounds like "relativism", but has none of the "there is no truth to be found . . . 'true' is just a name for what a bunch of people can agree on" implications of "relativism".[90]

There are, then, constraints on our conceptions of reality. Drawing my support from Putnam but staying with my own terminology, I call these "plausibility" and "coherence" constraints.

Plausibility Constraints in the philosophical literature are variously termed "operational," "natural," and "pragmatic" constraints or "action beliefs." Putnam refers to "experiential" constraints. They place limits on which conceptual systems will actually succeed, given the world that our minds and the world have jointly made up. Two examples from Putnam will suffice to make the point. He describes a conceptual system in which persons deem themselves able to fly and seek to act on it by jumping out of a window: "They would, if they were lucky enough to survive, see the weakness of the latter view at once."[91] He elsewhere uses a more mundane but equally illustrative example. If we attempted to construe the world so that steel would dissolve in water as does sugar, "nature would show us our mistake."[92] Important to note here is that nature itself is always construed by our conceptual schemes and is not utterly mind-independent. In both examples, we are prompted to revise our construal of the world.

Two criticisms of the bishops' letter claim that it violates plausibility constraints. The first is that the bishops' response in effect calls for a "bluff" deterrent: possessing but not intending to use nuclear weapons. The bishops' position is argued to be implausible given the degree of democratic participation in policy formation in the United States. This, in my opinion, is Finnis, Boyle, and Grisez's most acute criticism of the letter. Deterrence in relatively open societies is necessarily a social or public act.[93] A bluff deterrent, which depends upon the utmost secrecy, would therefore not work. The nature of superpower rivalry would show us our mistake. The second criticism is precisely that the bishops do not sufficiently take into account the geopolitical context of the nuclear situation. Deterrence is necessary because of the threat of Soviet Marxism-Leninism. Too severe limitations on strategic doctrine make our deterrent implausible and Soviet aggression more likely.[94] This criticism is countered by the observation that a construal of what is going on solely in terms of East-West rivalry obscures the North-South political-economic implications of a world with nuclear weapons.[95]

These and similar experiential constraints, however presently debated, eventually accumulate to form the wisdom of the tradition, including the tradition's readings of what constitutes human nature, human flourishing, and a just political society. Putnam gives a philosophical account of how traditions accumulate:

> In ethics, for example, we start with judgments that individual acts are right or wrong, ("observation reports", so to speak) and we gradually formulate maxims (not exceptionless generalizations) based on

those judgments, often accompanied by reasons or illustrative examples, as for instance "Be kind to a stranger among you, because you know what it was like to be a stranger in Egypt" (a "low level generalization"). These maxims in turn affect and alter our judgment about individual cases, so that new maxims supplementing or modifying the earlier ones may appear. After thousands of years of this dialectic between maxims and judgments about individual cases, a philosopher may come along and propose a moral conception (a "theory"), which may alter both maxims and singular judgments and so on. The very same procedure may be found in all of philosophy (which is almost coextensive with theory of rationality).[96]

The key point for our understanding of plausibility here is that while there is an accumulated tradition which takes into consideration experiential constraints, our repertoire of judgments, maxims, and theories—and ultimately our understandings of human nature and human flourishing—must remain open-ended and resist being hardened into immutable principles. Plausibility allows openness and response to God's challenge without sacrificing philosophical rigor.

Coherence Constraints are often called "theoretical" constraints. As outlined earlier, coherence is a function of plausibility. It aids to illumine a plausible response. Briefly stated, the constraint is that an incoherent response will not likely be plausible. An example is Finnis, Boyle, and Grisez's call for unilateral disarmament. The position is incoherent because the absolute status of the prohibition against the intention to kill the innocent shifts our moral attention away from large dimensions of what is going on where innocent persons are threatened by the unilateral policy. As argued earlier, such a prescription is also implausible.

A frequently discussed coherence constraint, and one important for the responsive-magisterial approach, is that of *conservatism*. Putnam gives a minimalist definition of the term: "Do not accept a theory which requires giving up a great many previously accepted beliefs if an otherwise equally 'simple' theory is available which preserves those beliefs and agrees with observation."[97] This constraint is particularly important for addressing the anticipated criticism that the effect of responses feeding back into and revising principles will be an uncontrollable revisionism. The principle of conservatism (which, incidentally, is of necessity itself open—in theory—to revision) points up the fact that the more basic principles and doctrines of a tradition are to perdure. There is a deep presumption against revision. Again, this is a function of plausibility. Putnam argues that revision cannot be unlimited because then "we would no longer have a concept of anything we could call rationality."[98] Put in our terms, there would be no tradition to engage in the rational activity of response at all.

Plausibility assumes significant continuity of tradition, which, through response to varying problem-situations over time, provides the substantive content of the rather thinly constituted criteria of plausibility and coherence. The accumulated wisdom of the tradition informs us that what we mean by human nature and human flourishing is not going to be radically discontinuous with previous responses either to that particular problem-situation or to other problem-situations of a relevant sort. (I take this latter continuity to be the fundamental impetus behind Cardinal Bernardin's "consistent ethic of life," though my criticisms of inherited understandings of *consistency* are now clear.) I would go further to say that plausibility and coherence imply that our responses will not be radically discontinuous with those of other communities. Shared problem-situations and experiential constraints, coupled with the fact of overlapping communities (I am a member not just of my church but of other "publics" as well), make discourse between traditions possible. This position differs both from some of the recent accounts of narrative that hold that the discourses of different communities are radically incommensurate and from an unrevised natural law theory that insists that the source of consensus is the single, "correct" understanding of the moral order. Indeed, the responsibility approach allows for the possibility of responses which are equally plausible and coherent and yet are logically incompatible. Putnam argues that one of the attractive features of pragmatic realism is "that it allows the possibility of alternative right versions of the world."[99] Continuity is not the same as uniformity. The bishops are aware of this when they argue that the just-war and pacifist options are complementary. Each keeps the other from being distorted within the community.[100] Rationality as response allows for this complementarity.

In sum, then, the plausibility and coherence constraints imply a mixed theory of moral truth, involving significantly revised elements of philosophically inherited "correspondence" and "coherence" theories. Regarding the former, there is correspondence first of all only of the overall response to the problem-situation, not to individual statements on specific objects or to properties of a fully independent order. Second, if the term *correspondence* is to be accepted at all, it must be understood loosely and not as having response "mirror" or "copy" reality. Here, the metaphor of *fit* better describes the actuality. Third, in internal realism, the correspondence of response to problem-situation is only within a description or conceptual scheme. Putnam prefers to drop the term *correspondence* altogether. Regarding the revised coherence constraints, the basic point is that any plausible system must also be coherent, but that not *any* coherent description or theory is adequate. Coherent responses, being functions of plausibility, must not violate the experiential constraints of plausibility itself. Plausibility and coherence are therefore mutually reinforcing. "Pragmatic realism," it seems, best describes this philosophical orientation. While Putnam uses the language of "fittingness" rather than plausibility, the affinities are clear: "What makes a statement, or a whole system of statements—a theory or conceptual scheme—rationally acceptable is, in large part, its coherence and fit; coherence of 'theoretical' or less experiential beliefs with one another and with more experiential beliefs, and also coherence of experiential beliefs with theoretical beliefs." And later: "Truth is ultimate goodness of fit."[101]

Having now set out the rational activity of response in terms of its affinities with Niebuhr, its reconstitution as plausibility and coherence, and its likely philosophical commitments, I turn to its ecclesiological counterpart, the organizational activity of response, to complete our account of the responsive-magisterial approach.

The Organizational Activity of Response

At the outset of this article, I stated that method (mode of reasoning) and ecclesiology (understanding of authority) are linked because they constitute two dimensions—the conceptual and the organizational—of the activity of a community as it seeks to address issues of consequence to human life. The main point in the present section is this: with rationality as plausibility and coherence, the understanding of the authority of church documents shifts away from the primary stress on the possession of first truths by particular persons or offices, and toward authority as a social relationship of trust.[102] This conception of authority applies to both audiences addressed in the bishops' letter: the members of the Catholic tradition and the larger U.S. public. Trust in each case is based upon the wisdom of the tradition as expressed in the plausibility and coherence of the church documents. Joseph Komonchak refers to this as trust in the "capacity to provide reasoned grounds for a decision."[103] The difference between the two audiences of the bishops' letter is that for those persons who are participants in the ecclesial tradition, the "faithful," there is an initial presumption in favor of the document. This is because to participate in a tradition is, in part, to trust in its accumulated wisdom, in its reflection over time on issues of consequence to human life. Other "publics" do not begin with this presumption or trust but can assess the document in terms of its plausibility and coherence from the perspective of their own interpretations of what is going on.

The presumption in favor of the document on the part of the participants in the tradition is the ecclesiological counterpart of the theoretical principle of conservatism discussed above. But just as conservatism does not involve immunity from revision, presumption does not grant absolute authority to the statements in the document. Reasons must still be given for the claims. Authority as a social relationship of trust therefore sets a particular context for interpreting the much debated phrase in Catholic ecclesiological literature *religiosum voluntatis et intellectus obsequium,* "religious submission of mind and will."[104] Trust in the tradition involves no less than a readiness to submit to its wisdom, but also no more.

The authority relationship within the tradition conserves and develops the accumulated wisdom. It therefore has a teaching function, thus the term *magisterial* for this understanding of authority. I counterpose this with the "official" model of authority not to indicate that offices are unnecessary or cannot serve a magisterial function, but to point up the fact that when they are combined with a deductive understanding of reason which grants officeholders epistemological privilege to first principles and their implications, then a preoccupation with particular offices and their juridical function can obscure and sometimes obstruct the teaching and learning activity of the tradition as a whole. The community's attention then focuses away from the issues—the challenges—at hand. We can ill afford to lose sight of the problem of the possession and use of nuclear weapons.

The emphasis in the bishops' letter is clearly on the teaching rather than the juridical function of their office.[105] Moreover, their office is subsumed under the community's broader task of responding to the situation which confronts it: "The nuclear threat transcends religious, cultural, and national boundaries. To confront its danger requires all the resources reason and faith can muster. This letter is a contribution to a wider common effort, meant to call Catholics and all members of our political community to dialogue and specific decisions about this awesome question."[106] The bishops are also aware that the complex and changing circumstances in political, military, and technological life require them to be learners as well as teachers.[107] They therefore recognize that the laity and members of other traditions also have a teaching function: "We have had to examine, with the assistance of a broad spectrum of advisors of varying persuasions, the nature of existing and proposed weapons systems, the doctrines which govern their use, and the consequences of using them. We have consulted people who engage their lives in protest against the existing nuclear strategy of the United States, and we have consulted others who have held or do hold responsibility for this strategy. It has been a sobering and perplexing experience."[108] In the magisterial approach to ecclesiology, all persons are both teachers and learners.

An anticipated concern is that the dialogical emphasis of trust based on plausibility and coherence turns the church and its deliberation into a "debating club."[109] Here it needs to be pointed out that the authority relationship is asymmetrical.[110] The needs of the community and the requirements of responsiveness necessitate the differentiation of roles and therefore the formation of offices. The theological backings for such offices (e.g., apostolic succession) are here interpreted not as final warrants for ecclesiastical legitimacy but as a means of articulating the trust in the historically accumulated wisdom of the tradition. The language of "levels" of authority then refers to levels of trust established around certain sets of beliefs and claims of the community. The more perduring claims may be so central to the identity of the tradition that to consistently be at odds with them is to be at odds with the community itself. Certain statements can and do mark the limits of legitimate participation in a community.

This much said, the magisterial approach emphasizes that authority is a *relationship* among participants of the community as they seek to respond to what is going on around them. Plausibility and coherence bring the relationship of trust to the fore, rather than the status of one member of that relationship. This has two immediate implications. First, the demands for responsiveness from a community change, and therefore the precise requirements of trust must also. This means that the limits of legitimate participation in the community, while necessarily having continuity over time, have no fixed interpretation. Second, if persons in church offices repeatedly violate the trust in them to conserve and develop the wisdom of the tradition, they weaken the authority relationship and thus their status as spokespersons of the responsive and responding community. The office is lessened precisely when emphasis on its status, apart from the relationship which gives it purpose, directs the community's attention and energy away from the challenge at hand. The church then becomes, in the sense we have been describing throughout, unresponsive.

The Case for Plausibility and Coherence

At the outset of this article, I stated that my task is to argue that the complex nature of public life in general and the problem-situation of the possession and potential use of nuclear weapons in particular require members of religious institutions to reconsider their understanding of the reason and authority of their social documents. I have set up two possible alternatives for interpreting and writing such documents in the Roman Catholic tradition: the deductive-official model and the responsive-magisterial approach. With these options laid out, we can now compare them more directly. In order to do this, we turn again to the concerns of the deductive-official model discussed in section one. Chief among them is that statements on policy particulars when not stipulated by moral absolutes have certain negative side effects with regard to forming the consciences of the faithful and shaping the public debate. Specific judgments confuse the consciences of the faithful, implying to laypersons that the statements carry more authority than they actually do. The result is an individualism among the faithful, where "cafeteria Catholics" pick and choose from the teachings. The impact on the public debate is weakened because judgments on policy particulars make the church simply one institution among others. The religious institution loses its uniqueness. In so doing, it also loses its influence on other public institutions. These negative side effects are ultimately the result of the fact that policy statements not directly derived from moral absolutes lack the certainty and immutability of general principles and are therefore subject to informed disagreement.

The responsive-magisterial approach does not so thoroughly separate principles and specific statements because the two are interactive in the community's activity of response. As a result, there is no methodological prejudgment against addressing particulars. This does not mean that in every instance bishops must speak to specifics. Recall that both the bishops and Niebuhr argue that the fundamental contribution of religious institutions is the introduction of religious and moral *perspectives* to the public debate.[111] If these perspectives are already suitably articulated by institutionally represented communities in public discussions, there is no immediate need for churches to directly participate. But if such a contribution is necessary, then specific policy judgments—distinguished but not separated from general principles—are to be part of its full articulation.

It is also important to note that the methodological status of the effects of addressing particulars differs in each of the two approaches. For the deductive-official model, they are "negative side effects." The argument is that to consider them otherwise would entail "consequentialism." This is especially important to recognize if a particular judgment is taken to be derived from an absolute moral norm, as with unilateral disarmament for Finnis, Boyle, and Grisez. In this case, no matter what the effects on the religious tradition and broader public, the judgment stands because its determining principle is absolute. For the responsive-magisterial approach, these effects are interpreted as constitutive dimensions of what is going on. Otherwise, the community's activity is not in accordance with the whole of the problem-situation. The question of the effects of statements of particulars is therefore one not just of side effects but also of the responsiveness of the tradition to the problem of the possession and potential use of nuclear weapons. The consideration of effectiveness appropriate to the theologically construed ultimate context in moral deliberation on possible responses is not methodological anathema. On the contrary, the absence of such consideration prematurely delimits what is morally relevant, and is therefore irresponsible.

Keeping in mind these basic differences between the two approaches to the issue of specifics, I can now address their implications for the formation of the consciences of the faithful and the shaping of the public debate.

Forming the Consciences of the Faithful

Criticism: Addressing policy specifics confuses the faithful, leading them to think that church representatives have more authority than they in fact have in political affairs.

Response: It is rather that a great number of laypersons already are confused and that judgments on policy particulars highlight this problem. It is better that churches do address specifics when necessary and that they be clear on the authority of the statements. To counsel silence on policy particulars is only to perpetuate a confusion, because, in practice, levels of authority other than that of "binding" principles are not acknowledged.

The point can be pushed even further. The ecclesial articulation of plausible and coherent arguments not only can dispel lay confusion on the issue of authority but also can serve to demonstrate, in a representative way, how moral arguments are made. The church here more adequately fulfills its teaching role—its function as *magister*—than when it passes over in silence the specifics of issues. The bishops insist: "To say 'no' to nuclear war is both a necessary and a complex task. We are moral teachers in a tradition which has always been prepared to relate moral principles to concrete problems. Particularly in this letter we could not be content with simply restating general moral principles or repeating well-known requirements about the ethics of war."[112]

Criticism: The responsive-magisterial approach leads to individualism and the phenomenon of "cafeteria Catholicism" because it implies that the faithful can pick and choose among teachings.

Response: This criticism is the ecclesiological counterpart to the charge of relativism. Again it does not hold. The responsive-magisterial approach emphasizes that it is the tradition as a whole that bears the accumulated wisdom and therefore the teaching function. Persons are to have a deep presumption that the teachings of the tradition, developed over time in response to a wide range of problem-situations, are true and right. I suggest that it is, at least in U.S. Catholicism, the deductive-official model that leads to individualism. This is because the tradition is so identified with particular offices, and not with the body of the faithful, and because such certainty is ascribed to the pronouncements of such offices (only "binding" principles and absolute moral judgments deducible from them may be articulated in documents) that when persons do dissent, the only sphere left for them to do so is that of an individual's own conscience. If there is no public means for dissent within the tradition, then unresolved issues become occasions for "private" dissent. Trust in the tradition then erodes, and individualism ensues.

The deductive-official model's emphasis on isolating immutable principles, which in fact are crystallizations of the community's responses to previous situations, itself exhibits a deep *dis*trust in the ability of the living tradition to address, through conserving and developing its accumulated wisdom, the present problems of human life. The stress is on avoiding guilt through obeying principles, and it is this that leads to an understanding of the conscience as a private matter. Niebuhr is to the point in describing the person who acts first of all in accordance with principles or laws, as opposed to responding to what is going on in light of the wisdom of the tradition:

> This man lives as moral self in the presence of law first of all, not of other selves. What is over against him is a commandment, a demand, a requirement. His relation to other selves is a relation under the law. They may be representatives of the law, enforcers of the law, or in their obedience to it may command respect; but his first relation is to the law and not to other persons. Hence when I understand myself with this idea in mind my conscience appears to me to be the center of the self. I decide in so defining the self that I will respect the conscience in myself and others as the most valuable element in selfhood, but the knowledge present in this conscience is knowledge of law and myself in relation to the law, not knowledge of other selves, or myself in relation to those selves.[113]

One reason why the deductive model of reasoning has become resistant to the reformulation of its principles is precisely that historically it has been combined—not without a great deal of tension between the two—with the understanding of authority as official. The principles of deductive reason are theoretically open to anyone's discernment. In practice, this leads to diversity. Uniformity is therefore brought about by closely identifying right reason with particular offices, and not with the tradition as a whole. Margaret Farley comments, "It is difficult not to be struck by a historical irony: a tradition that has never really repudiated a central role for human reason (in 'making sense' of the moral life) has nonetheless pushed toward an extrinsic authority (the hierarchical teaching office) as the ultimate source of each person's moral understanding."[114] Again, the analysis of the present article suggests that resistance to reformulation in the deductive model is closely linked to the understanding of authority as exclusively "official." The two are mutually reinforcing. Dissenting voices are left with no recognized forum except that of the private conscience.

From a responsive-magisterial perspective, it is important to note that one tack sometimes taken by persons in authority positions who accept the deductive-official view is to attempt to silence those who publicly articulate their dissent with regard to generally accepted teachings. In any elaboration of the effects of actions by the ecclesial community, the implications of silencing and its impact on trust within the community need to be taken into account as part of what is going on.[115]

Shaping the Public Debate

Criticism: Making prudential judgments on policy particulars threatens the uniqueness of the church by extending its discourse beyond theological doctrine and philosophical first principles.

Response: The problem stated here has merit as a general concern but not as a conclusive criticism. There is indeed a risk that religious institutions will lose their uniqueness if they address specifics. But it is just that: a risk. In contrast, the negative effects of not speaking to particulars when needed are all but given. This point needs elaboration.

As stated earlier, both Niebuhr and the bishops are in agreement that the fundamental contribution of religious institutions to public debates on policy issues is that of introducing a broad, theologically construed perspective. Such a perspective expands the scope of the morally relevant whole to be taken into account in the interpretation of what is going on. Most important for the nuclear debate, the theological context relativizes the East-West geopolitical construal of the situation while still allowing for relative judgments about the good and evil of each regime. In terms Niebuhr develops in *Radical Monotheism and Western Culture,* in a strategic debate where the tendency is toward henotheism—the absolutizing of finite communities—the bishops introduce a monotheistic perspective where only God is God.[116] This is the rebuttal against those who think that the bishops do not take geopolitical considerations seriously. While such considerations are important, they are not ultimate. For this reason, the bishops could never affirm Michael Walzer's argument for deterrence as a "supreme emergency" necessary to protect (Western) civilization.[117] Whatever arguments there may be for deterrence, however strictly conditioned, must be articulated in other terms.

Thus far, the deductive-official proponent has little to be concerned about. But the responsive-magisterial approach goes on to insist that what is at stake is not only the theological doctrines and general philosophical principles of a tradition, but also how these doctrines and principles cohere with the policy and practice of the community itself. Niebuhr argues well in *The Social Sources of Denominationalism* that distinctively Christian theological claims often mask the degree to which the social practices of the church reflect those of other institutions in the general public, including the practices of racism, nationalism, and economic injustice.[118] Refraining from specifics is therefore no safeguard against undesirable assimilation into the culture. More pointedly, it is only through the self-reflective process of connecting theological construals of life to the actual concrete practices of the church and its members in their professions that any uniqueness can be fostered and preserved. The bishops are aware of this fact when they write: "The Church is called to be, in a unique way, the instrument of the kingdom of God in history. Since peace is one of the signs of that kingdom present in the world, the Church fulfills part of her essential mission by making the peace of the kingdom more *visible* in our time" (emphasis added).[119] They realize that stating only theological doctrines and philosophical principles is insufficient.[120]

There is certainly a risk that in the working out of specifics in a public context full of immediate institutional exigencies, the church members will lose sight of the theological context. This has been one criticism leveled against Protestant church documents.[121] However, a theological doctrine severed from the real practice of its community not only threatens the uniqueness of the tradition, but works to veil this threat. The church is in this instance unique in word only. The problem then is that the church representation of the religious and moral perspective needed in public discourse is, at best, incomplete. At worst, it is hypocritical.

Criticism: In moving to policy particulars, and thus losing its uniqueness, the church loses its ability to influence other public institutions.

Response: On the contrary, when ecclesial institutions make plausible and coherent arguments which enter into the public debate, this obliges other institutions to do likewise. The Reagan administration felt it had to respond to drafts of the bishops' letter.[122] Strategists did as well.[123] The effect of this process of institutions, prompted by a church social document, attempting to articulate plausible and coherent arguments is a public which is more likely to "reason right" and act moderately. For the religious institution, which has traditionally sought restraint on the use of force, this must be considered a positive effect. In contrast, the restriction of church documents to general principles often has the effect that those very principles are self-interestedly misconstrued by other institutions. A full argument, which includes specifics, works to prevent this from happening.

It is, of course, sometimes the case that church documents are implausible and incoherent. The frequency of such occurrences prompts the kind of judgments, mentioned earlier, that Finnis makes concerning what he considers to be errors in the bishops' letter. They are the errors of "outsiders," who, by their very position in society, cannot make "truly prudential" judgments. By implication, government officials, the "insiders," do not make such mistakes.[124]

The problem with this account of the situation is that it is not at all clear that persons in government are always in the best position to make truly prudential judgments. There is considerable pressure during reelection campaigns. There is a tendency to make trade-offs based on localized interests in major bills on the Senate floor. In short, much policy is determined by factors having little to do with the prudential application of moral principles. It seems that, given the amount of nonclassified information that is available and especially given the time that the bishops spent in their open consultative process, there are cases in which the alleged outsider might be in a better position than the insider to make long-term prudential judgments on policy. The input of a major public institution less politically invested in a policy issue than are members of government can then have a positive effect. In any case, the plausibility and coherence of such input must be assessed in public exchange and must not be prejudged according to categories of insider/outsider status.

The suggestion that members of government are the only ones who are in the position to make truly prudential judgments is—depending on how far the suggestion is pushed—at least in tension with the idea of a democratic society, and at most incompatible with it. If not only bishops, but also columnists, teachers, lawyers—in short, all citizens—are by vocational definition deemed to be outsiders and therefore unable to make truly prudential judgments, then an uncritical attitude is fostered that would have an extremely negative effect on society.

The fact that various public institutions and communities have felt and still do feel compelled to respond to the argument of the bishops is no accident. The criteria of plausibility and coherence apply to any public institution desiring authority based on trust. This is especially the case in democratic societies. Recognizing the real differences in the way that authority is functionally structured in various "publics," we find that the understanding of authority as trust based on plausibility and coherence that is used to analyze ecclesial structures is sufficiently general to critique, on a case-by-case basis, the full array of social institutions. A religious institution putting forth plausible and coherent statements places the burden on public officials to do likewise, and not to rely simply on their official status to proclaim policy. This is no guarantee of agreement on issues, but it can at once both catalyze and temper discussion.

The above responses to criticisms are sufficient to indicate that the responsive-magisterial approach, when carried through plausibly and coherently, does not entail the negative effects outlined by the deductive-official model. Indeed, this latter model has disconcerting negative effects of its own. The import of these effects for the response approach is, once again, crucial if our deliberation is not to prematurely delimit what is morally relevant. The deductive-official model is unresponsive to what is going on in both the church community and wider society.

Conclusion

From the perspective of the response approach, there are clear methodological and historical reasons for the unresponsiveness of the deductive-official model. Principles, methods, and systems of thought arise as heuristic devices to aid the community in its rational and organizational activity of response, and they are legitimate to the degree that they continue to serve this function. The social document is a relatively new form of ecclesial literature, beginning in the late nineteenth century with the writings of Leo XIII. Such documents did not even explicitly address the broader public until Pius XII. The understanding of reason and authority in the deductive-official model was developed from the seventeenth to the first half of the twentieth century primarily as a means of weighing the severity of sins in the sacrament of penance—thus the emphasis on avoiding guilt. For this limited ecclesial function, the deductive approach offered a high degree of precision. The social document, in contrast, does not have the weighing of sins as its primary purpose. More, it functions in a sphere of human life where precision and certainty are difficult at best to attain.

The responsive-magisterial model aims to address problem-situations that are by their nature complex and often subject to rapid change. The deductive approach, as pointed out several times, is more closed to complexity and change. This sometimes results in responses which are implausible and coherent, and therefore irrational. The absolutist deductive argument for immediate unilateral disarmament has been our primary example. Given the degree of complexity and change in the problem-situations that social documents seek to address, the responsive-magisterial aim of the continuity and perdurability of the tradition is more adequate than the deductive-official ideal of the universality and immutability of particular principles. The responsive-magisterial approach is more efffective as a way to critique and compose social documents because its very aim is to be responsive to the problem-situations which such documents seek to address. What is at stake is nothing less than our responsibility to and for God's challenge in the problem-situation of the possession and potential use of nuclear weapons.

Notes

1. Stephen Toulmin, *Human Understanding: The Collective Use and Evolution of Concepts* (Princeton: Princeton University Press, 1972), 501–2.

2. The issue of the implications of the responsive-magisterial approach for Protestant denominations arose in the discussion of this essay at the 1988 meeting of the American Academy of Religion. While it cannot be argued in detail here, I think that the responsive-magisterial approach offers the emphasis on perduring tradition that is necessary to make a response to large social problems possible without violating the centrality of the person's conscience that is the mark of much of Protestant ethics.

3. National Conference of Catholic Bishops, *The Challenge of Peace: God's Promise and Our Response* (Washington, D.C.: United States Catholic Conference, 1983).

4. This is not to say that the only important criticisms of the bishops' letter are from the deductive-official approach. In fact, the argument in part is that the responsive-magisterial model provides a more adequate basis on which to critique *The Challenge of Peace* and other documents.

5. "Rome Consultation on Peace and Disarmament: A Vatican Synthesis," *Origins* 12 (April 7, 1983): 691–95.

6. Ibid., 692, 693, 695.

7. Ibid., 693, 695.

8. Ibid., 693.

9. John Finnis, "The Consistent Ethic of Life: A Philosophical Critique," prepared for the Symposium on the Consistent Ethic of Life, Loyola University of Chicago, November 7, 1987, p. 5. At the time of this writing, the papers of the conference are being prepared for publication by Sheed and Ward in the fall of 1988. My page references shall therefore be to the conference paper.

10. Ibid., 6.

11. Ibid., 7.

12. Ibid.

13. Ibid., 7–8.

14. Ibid., 14.

15. Ibid., 31, 33.

16. Ibid., 34–43, 44–50, 66–67 n. 64.

17. John Finnis, Joseph M. Boyle, Jr., and Germain Grisez, *Nuclear Deterrence, Morality, and Realism* (Oxford: Clarendon Press, 1987), 177, 283ff., quote on 291.

18. Ibid., 161. Cf. also 200, 283; and Finnis, "Consistent Ethic of Life," 44.

19. Finnis, "Consistent Ethic of Life," 25.

20. *The Challenge of Peace*, par. 28; cf. also pars. 276, 331, 333, where the language of promise/challenge and response is articulated in terms of gift/call and response.

21. For treatments of the philosophical and theological development of the term *responsibility,* see Richard McKeon, "The Development and the Significance of the Concept of Responsibility," *Revue internationale de philosophie* 34 (1957): 3–32; and Albert R. Jonsen, *Responsibility in Modern Religious Ethics* (Washington, D.C.: Corpus Books, 1968).

22. See Martin Buber, *I and Thou,* trans. Walter Kaufmann (New York: Charles Scribner's Sons, 1970); Dietrich Bonhoeffer, *Ethics* (New York: Macmillan, 1955), 188–262; Bernard Häring, *The Law of Christ,* vol. I (Westminster, Md.: Newman Press, 1961), 35–213; Robert Johann, *Building the Human* (New York: Mentor-Omega, 1967); H. Richard Niebuhr, *The Responsible Self* (New York: Harper and Row, 1963). Excerpts of the writings of various authors on the topic of responsibility are brought together in a helpful way in James M. Gustafson and James T. Laney, eds., *On Being Responsible: Issues in Personal Ethics* (New York: Harper and Row, 1968).

23. Niebuhr, *The Responsible Self,* 46, 60, 56; cf. also 59, 94.

24. Ibid., 60–65.

25. James M. Gustafson, Introduction to Niebuhr, *The Responsible Self,* 8.

26. Niebuhr, *The Responsible Self,* 126, 61.

27. It is noteworthy that Bernard Häring also uses the language of "fitting" and again in the normative as well as descriptive sense: "Hence, we understand Christian morality as responsibility in the sense that the Christian in his relationship to himself, to his human co-world, to the world of creatures, perceives a word and message which ultimately comes from God. This responsibility further requires that in his thinking, speaking and acting, in his personal relationships, and in shaping the world he give a fitting reply, that he act responsibly and so much so that everything in the last analysis becomes a reply, a response that is worthy to be offered to God." Häring, "Religion and Morality: Fellowship and Responsibility," in *Personalism in Philosophy and Theology,* 12, cited in Jonsen, *Modern Religious Ethics,* 92.

28. *The Challenge of Peace*, pars. 1–3; see also pars. 13 and 125 (the "signs of the times") and 126–38 (the "new moment") for further descriptions of "what is going on."

29. Niebuhr, *The Responsible Self,* 59.

30. See, for instance, *The Challenge of Peace*, par. 122.

31. Ibid., pars. 27–65.

32. Niebuhr, *The Responsible Self,* 107.

33. *The Challenge of Peace*, par. 161.

34. Ibid., pars. 17, 32–38, 44–51, 54–55.

35. For the language of *vision* and *image,* see ibid., pars. 20, 25, 32, 34, 36, 38, 58, 67, 131, 134, 202, 303.

226   Whitmore

36. Ibid., par. 28; for the language of *in light of,* see also pars. 2, 8, 13, 32, 132, 190–91.

37. I am indebted to James M. Gustafson for this observation. See his "The Bishops' Pastoral Letter: A Theological Ethical Analysis," *Criterion* 23, no. 2 (Spring 1984): 5–10. See also "The Relation of the Church to the War in Light of the Christian Faith," *Social Action* 10, no. 10 (December 15, 1944). The commission, more commonly called the "Calhoun Commission," also included Robert Lowry Calhoun, Roland Bainton, John C. Bennett, and Reinhold Niebuhr among its members. For H. Richard Niebuhr's own reflections on war in light of the Christian faith, see his "War as the Judgment of God," *Christian Century* 59, no. 19 (May 13, 1942): 630–33; "Is God in the War?" *Christian Century* 59, no. 31 (August 5, 1942): 953–55; and "War as Crucifixion," *Christian Century* 60, no. 17 (April 28, 1943): 513–15. For a helpful analysis of how Niebuhr's war articles relate to his thought as a whole, see Richard B. Miller, "H. Richard Niebuhr's War Articles: A Transvaluation of Value," *Journal of Religion* 68, no. 2 (April 1988): 242–62.

38. *The Challenge of Peace,* par. 55; see also par. 29. One of the criticisms of the pastoral letter is that it does not sufficiently integrate the theological language of response with the middle sections of the document. See Gustafson, "The Bishops' Pastoral Letter," 6–7; and Sandra M. Schneiders, "New Testament Reflections on Peace and Nuclear Arms," in Philip J. Murnion, ed., *Catholics and Nuclear War: A Commentary on "The Challenge of Peace"* (New York: Crossroad, 1983), 91–105.

39. Ibid., pars. 4 (see also par. 24), 26, 230, 195, 276.

40. Ibid., pars. 21, 4, 6, 12, 23, 129–30, 132, 139, 141, 152, 195–96, 220, 230, 329.

41. For an account of the bishops' consultative process, see Jim Castelli, *The Bishops and the Bomb* (New York: Image Books, 1983).

42. For example, see Michael Novak, "Example of Open Church in Practice," *National Catholic Reporter* (April 22, 1983); and James E. Dougherty, *The Bishops and Nuclear Weapons* (Cambridge, Mass.: Archon Books, 1984), 127–28.

43. *The Challenge of Peace,* par. 5; see also par. 328.

44. Ibid.; for the theological context of peace, see pars. 27–65; for the political order, pars. 66–79; for the use of force, pars. 80–121. This progression from theology to political theory to the use of force counters George Weigel's charge that the bishops do not place the just-war tradition within the context of teachings about right political order. After a treatment of fundamental political concepts, and before detailing the just-war criteria, the bishops give us the following transitional paragraph: "In light of the framework of Catholic teaching on the nature of peace, the avoidance of war, and the state's right of legitimate defense, we can now spell out certain moral principles within the Catholic tradition which provide guidance for public policy and individual choice" (par. 79). Pars. 234–73 also discuss the political context of Catholic teaching on world order. See Weigel, *Tranquillitas Ordinis: The Present Failure and Future Promise of American Catholic Thought on War and Peace* (Oxford: Oxford University Press, 1987), 257–80. For the bishops' use of the *Pastoral Constitution on the Church in the Modern World* in *The Challenge of Peace,* see pars. 7, 62–65.

45. Jonsen, *Modern Religious Ethics,* 206. Jonsen cites par. 55 of the *Pastoral Constitution:* "In every group or nation, there is an ever-increasing number of men and women who are conscious that they themselves are the artisans and the authors of the culture of their community. Throughout the world there is a similar growth in the combined sense of independence and responsibility. Such a development is of paramount importance for the spiritual and moral maturity of the human race. . . . We are witnesses of the birth of a new humanism, one in which man is defined first by his responsibility toward his brothers and toward history."

46. Niebuhr, *The Responsible Self,* 96.

47. Jonsen writes concerning a responsibility ethic, "A rule is morally valid when it directs us back to the reality from which it was drawn and focuses our attention and decision upon the values demanded by the reality." Jonsen, *Modern Religious Ethics,* 205.

48. See Niebuhr, *The Responsible Self,* 56–57, 62–63. Both McKeon and Jonsen argue that the response approach unifies without eliminating teleology and deontology. See McKeon, "Concept of Responsibility," 32; and Jonsen, *Modern Religious Ethics,* 183.

49. *The Challenge of Peace,* pars. 147–49, 150–61.

50. See Leroy Walters, "Five Classic Just War Theories: A Study in the Thought of Thomas Aquinas, Vitoria, Suarez, Gentili, and Grotius" (Ph.D. diss., Yale University, 1971); and James T. Johnson, *Just War Tradition and the Restraint of War: A Moral and Historical Inquiry* (Princeton: Princeton University Press, 1981).

51. *The Challenge of Peace,* par. 28.

52. Ibid., par. 14.

53. For a treatment of the types of discourse, see James M. Gustafson, *Varieties of Moral Discourse: Prophetic, Narrative, Ethical, and Policy* (Grand Rapids, Mich.: Calvin College and Seminary, 1988).

54. Bernard Häring accounts for the possibility through his understanding of "historicity," which is part of the "constitutive structure" of the human person. See Häring, "Dynamism and Continuity in a Personalistic Approach to Natural Law," in Gene Outka and Paul Ramsey, eds., *Norm and Context in Christian Ethics* (New York: Scribner, 1968), 203.

55. *The Challenge of Peace,* par. 122; cf. also pars. 124–25.

56. Ibid., par. 304; also par. 24: "A fresh reappraisal which includes a developed theology of peace will require contributions from several sectors of the Church's life: biblical studies, systematic and moral theology, ecclesiology, and the experience and insights of members of the Church who have struggled in various ways to make and keep the peace in this often violent age. This pastoral letter is more an invitation to continue the new appraisal of war and peace than a final synthesis of the results of such an appraisal. We have some sense of the characteristics of a theology of peace, but not a systematic statement of their relationships."

57. For a historical treatment of the loss of the context of peace in just-war thought and a call for its retrieval, see J. T. Delos, "The Sociology of Modern War and the Theory of Just War," *Cross Currents* 8, no. 3 (Summer 1958): 248–66. Once again this evidences that the bishops are retrieving rather than abandoning the tradition. See n. 44 above.

58. Pius XII, "Christmas Message, 1956," in Vincent A. Yzermans, ed., *The Major Addresses of Pope Pius XII,* vol. II (St. Paul, Minn.: North Central Publishing Co., 1961), 225.

59. *Pastoral Constitution on the Church in the Modern World,* pars. 78–79, in Walter M. Abbott, S.J., ed., *The Documents of Vatican II* (Piscataway, N.J.: America Press, 1966), 290–93; and National Conference of Catholic Bishops, *Human Life in Our Day* (Washington, D.C.: United States Catholic Conference, 1968), 44. *The Challenge of Peace* cites these documents in par. 118.

60. *The Challenge of Peace,* pars. 73–74, 120–21, 60–62.

61. David Hollenbach, S.J., "*The Challenge of Peace* in the Context of Recent Church Teachings," in Murnion, *Catholics and Nuclear War,* 6–8; and Francis X. Meehan, "NonViolence and the Bishops' Pastoral: A Case for the Development of Doctrine," in Judith A. Dwyer, ed., *The Catholic Bishops and Nuclear War* (Washington, D.C.: Georgetown University Press, 1984). See Duane K. Friesen's article in this volume. James Finn argues that the development of a view that just war and pacifism are complementary

"corrupts" both traditions. See his "Pacifism and Just War: Either or Neither," in Murnion, *Catholics and Nuclear War,* 142–45.

62. It needs to be noted here that the presumption against war that the bishops highlight has not always been present in just-war thought. See Delos, "Theory of Just War." For the bishops' discussion of this presumption, see *The Challenge of Peace,* pars. 70, 80–84.

63. *The Challenge of Peace,* pars. 88–90 (on competent authority); 96–97 (on last resort); 101 (on noncombatant immunity and proportionality); 92–94, 186–88.

64. David Hollenbach, S.J., *Nuclear Ethics: A Christian Moral Argument* (New York: Paulist Press, 1983), 75.

65. *The Challenge of Peace,* pars. 8–11.

66. For an interpretation of the bishops as following a deductive approach, see Charles Curran, "The Moral Methodology of the Bishops' Pastoral," in Murnion, *Catholics and Nuclear War,* 53ff. For the argument that the bishops do not follow in practice the strict universal principle/specific application, see William E. Murnion, "The Role and Language of the Church in Relation to Public Policy," in idem, 61ff.

67. Ibid., pars. 104, 15.

68. For a collection of essays on double effect, see Charles E. Curran and Richard A. McCormick, S.J., eds., *Readings in Moral Theology, No. 1: Moral Norms and the Catholic Tradition* (New York: Paulist Press, 1979).

69. Paul Ramsey, *War and the Christian Conscience* (Durham, N.C.: Duke University Press, 1961).

70. See Finnis, Boyle, and Grisez, *Nuclear Deterrence,* 160–61; Joseph M. Boyle, Jr., "*The Challenge of Peace* and the Morality of Nuclear Deterrence," in Charles J. Reid, Jr., ed., *Peace in a Nuclear Age: The Bishops' Pastoral Letter in Perspective* (Washington, D.C.: Catholic University of America Press, 1986), 323–35; David A. Hoekema, "Morality, Just War, and Nuclear Weapons: An Analysis of *The Challenge of Peace,*" *Soundings* 67 (1984); François Gorand, "La dissuasion nucleaire," *Etudes* (October 1983), 377–88; Charles Krauthammer, "On Nuclear Morality," *Commentary* (October 1983), 48–52; Susan Moller Okin, "Taking the Bishops Seriously," *World Politics* 36 (1984): 527–54; *New Yorker,* editorial (May 23, 1983), 31–32; Robert Roth, S.J., "Nuclear Deterrence and the Bishops' Pastoral Letter," *Thought* 59 (1987): 15–24; Bruce M. Russett, "The Doctrine of Deterrence," in Murnion, *Catholics and Nuclear War,* 149–68; Albert Wohlstetter, "Bishops, Statesmen, and Other Strategists on the Bombing of Innocents," *Commentary* (June 1983), 15–35; and John Howard Yoder in this volume.

71. Finnis, Boyle, and Grisez, *Nuclear Deterrence,* 161.

72. Ibid., 334–35.

73. Again, Jonsen writes that in a responsibility ethic, "A rule is morally valid when it directs . . . our attention and decision upon the values demanded by the reality." Jonsen, *Modern Religious Ethics,* 205. Finnis, Boyle, and Grisez's use of the principle of no direct killing of innocents directs attention away from the value it seeks to protect.

74. *The Challenge of Peace,* pars. 28, 83, 64, 122.

75. Ladislas Orsy, S.J., writes, "The absence of orderly procedures (for change) is one of the reasons why the Catholic Church suffers so frequently from internal agitations and conflicts; they appear to the faithful as the only means of bringing to the notice of the authorities that some measure of change is needed." See his "Magisterium: Assent and Dissent," *Theological Studies* 48 (1987): 473.

76. See McKeon, "Concept of Responsibility," 31.

77. *The Challenge of Peace,* pars. 17, 71.

78. Häring, *Law of Christ.*

79. See Outka and Ramsey, *Christian Ethics,* for a good collection of representative articles on this debate. There was also an earlier Roman Catholic "situation ethics" debate in the 1940s and 1950s. Pius XI condemned the movement in 1952. It was censured by the Holy Office in 1956. See John C. Ford, S.J., and Gerald Kelly, S.J., *Contemporary Moral Theology,* vol. 1 (Westminster, Md.: Newman Press, 1958), 104–40; and Robert W. Gleason, "Situational Morality," *Thought* 32 (1957): 533–58.

80. For well-written articles that help sort out the confusion, see Lisa Sowle Cahill, "Contemporary Challenges to Exceptionless Moral Norms," in *Moral Theology Today: Certitudes and Doubts* (St. Louis: Pope John XXIII Center, 1984), 121–35; and Edward Vacek, S.J., "Proportionalism: One View of the Debate," *Theological Studies* 46, no. 2 (Summer 1985).

81. Finnis, Boyle, and Grisez, *Nuclear Deterrence,* 181–82, 195–201.

82. Ibid., v, 251–52.

83. W. D. Ross, *The Right and the Good* (Oxford: Clarendon, 1930), ch. 2. For an analysis of just-war norms in terms of prima facie duties, see James F. Childress, "Just War Criteria," in Thomas A. Shannon, ed., *War or Peace? The Search for New Answers* (Maryknoll, N.Y.: Orbis, 1980), 40–58.

84. Morton White, *What Is and What Ought to Be Done: An Essay on Ethics and Epistemology* (New York and Oxford: Oxford University Press, 1981), esp. ch. 3.

85. Ibid.; see, for instance, 60, 66.

86. Hilary Putnam, *Reason, Truth, and History* (Cambridge: Cambridge University Press, 1981); *Realism and Reason: Philosophical Papers,* vol. 3 (Cambridge: Cambridge University Press, 1983); and *The Many Faces of Realism* (LaSalle, Ill.: Open Court, 1987). In the earlier two books, Putnam uses the term *internal realism.* In the last book, he goes back and forth between this and *pragmatic realism* but clearly prefers the latter term: "The key to working out the program of preserving commonsense realism . . . is something I have called *internal realism.* (I should have called it pragmatic realism!)" (17).

87. It seems to me that persons within the Roman Catholic tradition who talk about the horizons of knowledge hold an epistemology compatible with internal realism. Note this passage from Ladislas Orsy: "Horizons can never be bridged by dialogue alone, since the meaning of the words depends not only on its content but on its place within a given horizon. (The same words can carry different meanings in different horizons.) . . . The passage from one horizon to another is never through conceptual understanding; it is a surrender of the whole person to a new environment." Orsy, "Magisterium," 494 n. 37.

88. Putnam, *Reason, Truth, and History,* 49.

89. Ibid., xi; restated in Putnam, *The Many Faces of Realism,* 1.

90. Putnam, *The Many Faces of Realism,* 17–18.

91. Putnam, *Reason, Truth, and History,* 54.

92. Putnam, *The Many Faces of Realism,* 31.

93. Finnis, Boyle, and Grisez, *Nuclear Deterrence,* 113–23; Yoder also makes this observation in this volume.

94. The persons who make this criticism are many. In one volume on the bishops' letter, there are five essays setting forth this position: Michael Novak, "Realism, Dissuasion, and Hope in the Nuclear Age," 123–26; Edward N. Luttwak, "Catholics and the Bomb: The Perspective of the Non-Catholic Strategist," 159–70; George Weigel, "The Bishops' Pastoral Letter and American Political Culture: Who Was Influencing Whom?" 171–89; Vin Weber, "Revisionist History: A Catholic Perspective on the Nuclear Freeze Movement," 190–207; and Robert R. Reilly, "In Proportion to What? The Problem with the Pastoral," 208–26; all in Reid, *Peace in a Nuclear Age.*

95. See Peter J. Henriot, S.J., "Disarmament and Development: The Lasting Challenge to Peace," in ibid., 227-37.

96. Putnam, *Reason, Truth, and History,* 104-5; cf. also 134.

97. Ibid., 31; see also White, *What Is,* 64-65, 75, esp. 93: "Although I refrain from using the notions of meaning and essence, I think I understand and sympathize with the intentions of some philosophers who employ these notions. Keeping these intentions in mind, I am quite prepared to grant that we are properly more reluctant to surrender some statements that figure in certain conjunctions than we are to surrender others, and that what are called analytic statements or essential truths coincide to some extent with those statements that we have a right or duty to protect to the bitter end in any inquiry."

98. Putnam, *Reason, Truth, and History,* 83-84.

99. Cf. ibid., 73, 79.

100. *The Challenge of Peace,* pars. 60-62.

101. Ibid., 54-55, 64.

102. For discussions of ecclesial authority in terms of trust, see Joseph Komonchak, "Authority and Magisterium," in William W. May, ed., *Vatican Authority and American Catholic Dissent: The Curran Case and Its Consequences* (New York: Crossroad, 1987), 103-14; and Edward Schillebeeckx, "The Magisterium and Ideology," 5-17, and Franz-Xaver Kaufmann, "The Sociology of Knowledge and the Problem of Authority," 18-31, both in Leonard Swidler and Piet F. Fransen, *Authority in the Church and the Schillebeeckx Case* (New York: Crossroad, 1982).

103. Komonchak, "Authority and Magisterium," 110.

104. The phrase appears in the Second Vatican Council document *Lumen Gentium,* par. 25, in Abbott, *The Documents of Vatican II,* 47-50. For solid treatments of the concept of *obsequium,* see Francis J. Sullivan, S.J., *Magisterium: Teaching Authority in the Catholic Church* (Dublin: Gill and MacMillan, 1983); and Ladislas Orsy, S.J., *The Church: Learning and Teaching* (Wilmington, Del.: Michael Glazier, Inc., 1987), 82-89.

105. *The Challenge of Peace,* pars. 132, 139-41.

106. Ibid., par. 6; cf. also pars. 21, 139 ("We see our role as moral teachers precisely in terms of helping to form public opinion with a clear determination to resist resort to nuclear war as an instrument of national policy"), 141 ("We believe religious leaders have a task in concert with public officials, analysts, private organizations, and the media to set the limits beyond which our military policy should not move in word or action"), 230, 329.

107. For treatments of a teaching/learning ecclesiology, see Richard A. McCormick, S.J., "Reflections on the Literature," in Charles E. Curran and Richard A. McCormick, S.J., *Readings in Moral Theology, No. 3: The Magisterium and Morality* (New York: Paulist Press, 1982), 461-510; and Orsy, *The Church.*

108. *The Challenge of Peace,* par. 132.

109. See, for instance, Archbishop Roger M. Mahoney, "The Magisterium and Theological Dissent," in May, *Vatican Authority,* 16-26.

110. Komonchak, "Authority and Magisterium," 103.

111. *The Challenge of Peace,* par. 161; and Niebuhr, *The Responsible Self,* 107.

112. *The Challenge of Peace,* par. 132.

113. Niebuhr, *The Responsible Self,* 70-71.

114. Margaret A. Farley, "Moral Discourse in the Public Arena," in May, *Vatican Authority,* 174.

115. For treatments of the impact of silencing on the church community, see ibid., 168-86; and Archbishop Rembert Weakland, O.S.B., "The Price of Orthodoxy," *Catholic Herald* (September 11 and 18, 1986).

116. H. Richard Niebuhr, *Radical Monotheism and Western Culture* (New York: Harper and Row, 1943).

117. See Michael Walzer, *Just and Unjust Wars: A Moral Argument with Historical Illustrations* (New York: Basic Books, Inc., 1977), 251–74.

118. H. Richard Niebuhr, *The Social Sources of Denominationalism* (New York: H. Holt and Co., 1929). One might add to racism, nationalism, and economic injustice the social practice of sexism as one which inflicts the church as well as the broader public.

119. *The Challenge of Peace*, par. 22.

120. See n. 112 above.

121. See Paul Ramsey, *Who Speaks for the Church?* (Nashville, Tenn.: Abingdon Press, 1967); and *Speak Up for Just War or Pacifism* (University Park: Pennsylvania State University Press, 1988). A notable exception to this trend in Protestant documents toward underdeveloped theological contexts is the Calhoun Commission document. See n. 37 above.

122. *The Challenge of Peace*, par. 179 n. 81.

123. See J. Bryan Hehir's article "Ethics and Strategy," in this volume.

124. Finnis, "Consistent Ethic of Life," 48 n. 64.

Notes on the Contributors

Duane K. Friesen is professor of Bible and religion at Bethel College, North Newton, Kansas. He is the author of *Christian Peacemaking and International Conflict: A Realist Pacifist Perspective*.

J. Bryan Hehir is counselor for social policy, the United States Catholic Conference. He is also senior research scholar, Kennedy Institute of Ethics, and research professor of ethics and international politics, Georgetown University. He was a staff consultant to the National Conference of Catholic Bishops Ad Hoc Committee on War and Peace in its writing of the pastoral letter *The Challenge of Peace*. He is the coauthor, with Robert Gessert, of *The New Nuclear Debate*.

David Hollenbach, S.J., is associate professor of moral theology, Weston School of Theology, Cambridge, Massachusetts. He is the author of *Nuclear Ethics: A Christian Moral Argument*.

James Turner Johnson is professor of religion at Rutgers University. He is the author of *Ideology, Reason, and the Limitation of War; Just War Tradition and the Restraint of War; Can Modern War Be Just?;* and *The Quest for Peace: Three Moral Traditions in Western Cultural History*.

John Langan, S.J., is Rose F. Kennedy Professor of Christian Ethics at the Kennedy Institute of Ethics, Georgetown University, and senior fellow at the Woodstock Theological Center. He is the coeditor, with William V. O'Brien, of *The Nuclear Dilemma and the Just War Tradition*.

Richard B. Miller is assistant professor of religious studies at Indiana University at Bloomington.

Trutz Rendtorff is on the Protestant Faculty of the Institute for Systematic Theology, University of Munich, Federal Republic of Germany.

He is the author of *Ethics: Basic Elements and Methodology in an Ethical Theology*.

Todd Whitmore is director of the Colloquium on Religion and World Affairs, University of Chicago.

John Howard Yoder is professor of theology at Goshen Seminary in Elkhart, Indiana, and at the University of Notre Dame. His books include *The Politics of Jesus, The Priestly Kingdom: Social Ethics and the Gospel, Nevertheless: The Varieties of Religious Pacifism,* and *When War Is Unjust: Being Honest in Just-War Thinking*.

Index

Accountability, 194
Adenauer, Konrad, 139
Alessi, Victor, 123
Anscombe, Gertrude, 85, 134
Aristotle, 52, 53, 54
Arms control, 28, 29, 31, 104, 114
Augustine, 70, 85, 150
Authority, 84-85; competent, 201; ecclesiastical, 5

Bainton, Roland, 161
Barbour, Ian, 173
Barth, Karl, theological influence of, 141
Bennett, John, 1
Bernardin, Joseph Cardinal, 123-24, 185, 212
Bluffing, 5, 41, 43, 47, 48, 80, 81, 82, 87, 90, 210
Bockle, Franz, 124
Bohr, Niels, 141, 173
Bok, Derek, 4
Bok, Sissela, 39
Bonhoeffer, Dietrich, 190
Boulding, Kenneth, 170
Boyle, Joseph, Jr., 187, 188, 203, 204, 206-8, 210, 211, 217
Bracken, Paul, 47
Brennan, Donald, 29
Brodie, Bernard, 151
Brown, Dale, 164
Brzezinski, Zbigniew, 30; strategy of, 27-28
Buber, Martin, 190
Bundy, McGeorge, 2, 26, 30; strategy of, 23-25

Carnegie Council on Ethics and International Affairs, 3
Carter administration, 25, 27, 125
Casaroli, Cardinal, 183, 184, 189, 199
Catholic bishops, French, 59, 64, 72; document of, 122
Catholic bishops, U.S., 37, 40, 75, 76, 82, 97, 101-2, 111, 121, 126, 129-37, 143, 147, 163, 169, 171-76, 182, 200; authority of, 185; conference of, 124, 183; document of, 123
Catholic bishops, West German, 60, 61, 64, 72, 127, 128; conference of, 124, 143; document of, 122, 123
Catholic Worker Movement, 121-22
CEP, 112, 113; low, 6, 108, 111, 115
The Challenge of Peace, 1-4, 14, 18, 23, 25, 27, 75, 82, 86, 97, 101, 121, 163, 182, 187, 189-91, 195, 200
Chernobyl disaster, 113
Childress, James, 1, 98
Christian pacifism. *See* Evangelical pacifism
Christian Peacemaking and International Conflict, 164, 174
Church of England, 122
Coherence, 195, 222-24; case for, 216-17; constraints on, 211-13; definition of, 198; philosophical considerations of, 205-9
Collateral damage, 71, 73, 75, 107, 108, 112, 114, 137
Command systems, strengthening, 19, 137
Commission for Public Responsibility, 142

Communication systems, improving, 75, 137

Competence de guerre, 97

Confessing Church, 141. See also *Status confessionis*

The Confession to Jesus Christ and the Responsibility of the Church for Peace, 143–44

Conscientious objection, 200

Consequentialism, 36, 79, 84, 86–88, 185, 205–8, 217

Control, improvements in, 137

Conventional war, 50, 60, 103, 147

Conventional weapons, 22, 25, 26, 40, 63, 74, 108, 111, 113, 114, 147

Convergence, 163, 177; definition of, 162

Correspondence, 212–23

Council of the Evangelical Church in Germany, 142

Council on Religion and International Affairs. *See* Carnegie Council on Ethics and International Affairs

Countercity targeting, 40–43, 45, 60, 100. *See also* Targeting policy

Counterforce targeting, 42, 45, 65, 71, 72, 73, 105, 108, 110, 112–14, 136

Counterpopulation targeting, 19, 63, 64, 101, 105, 108, 110, 112, 113, 197

Countervalue targeting, 73, 74, 110

Criminality, definition of, 62

Cruise missiles, 108, 125

Cuban missile crisis, 38

Curran, Charles, 124

Czempiel, Ernst-Otto, 124

Daugherty, James, 123

Decapitation strategy, 25, 73, 74

Deductive-official model, 181, 199, 216–20, 223, 224; inadequacy of, 182; summary of, 183–84

Defensive options, 28, 30, 31, 76

Deontology, 79, 129, 134, 190, 192, 196, 197, 206; rejection of, 3

Deterrence, 5, 11, 22, 29, 30, 37, 40–50, 53, 55, 59, 60, 65, 71, 73, 80–84, 87, 88, 90, 91, 96, 106, 112, 114, 115, 121, 125, 126, 128, 129, 131, 132, 134–39, 144, 146–49, 151, 152, 172,

175–77, 187, 188, 203, 208, 220; conditional acceptance of, 17–20, 23–27, 133; counterpopulation, 64; countervalue, 72; deterioration of, 38–39; ethical assessment of, 19, 99–103, 127; existential, 23–25; John Paul II and, 130; justification for, 14–15, 51; maximal, 74; minimal, 74–76; morality of, 35, 127, 130; objections to, 15–17; pacifism and, 167; problematic of, 6. *See also* Threat

Disarmament, 42, 44, 91, 111, 114, 126, 128, 129; unilateral, 188, 197, 203, 211, 217. *See also* Nuclear pacifism; Pacifism; Unilateralism

Discrimination, 6, 14, 21–23, 26, 27, 29, 40, 41, 67, 73, 80, 107, 108, 111, 112, 129, 130, 131, 135, 136

Distress: ethics of, 70; situation of, 59–65

Double effect, 91, 101, 102, 111, 129, 131, 202–3; doctrine of, 85

Dougherty, Edward, 124

Emergency system, 60

Escalation, 15, 16, 40, 44, 45, 71, 82, 87, 90, 125, 131, 132, 136, 137

Eschatology, 68–70, 142

Ethic of ends, 29–30

Ethic of means, 29–30

Ethics, 1, 13; distress and, 59; emergency, 60; limited war and, 71–76; nuclear strategy and, 14, 28–31; Protestant, 206

Eudaimonia, 53

Evangelical pacifism, 169, 171, 174–76; definition of, 164

Exceptionalist thesis, criticism of, 52–55

Farley, Margaret, 219

Federal Council of Churches, 193

Finn, James, 172

Finnis, John, 134, 185–88, 199, 203, 204, 206–8, 210, 211, 217, 222

First strike, 15, 81, 87, 105; counterforce, 40, 41, 43, 73; preemptive, 27; selective, 28

First use, 18, 19, 45, 131, 132, 136

Force de frappe, 60
Ford, John C., 1, 63
Fractional megatonnage, 95, 103, 111, 112, 115
Fraling, Bernard, 124
Freedman, Lawrence, 47, 63, 71, 73
Friesen, Duane K., 201

Gandhi, 165
Gannon, Thomas, 124
Gaudium et Spes. See Pastoral Constitution on the Church in the Modern World (Gaudium et Spes)
General Synod of the Churches in East Germany, 144
General Synod of the Evangelical Church in Germany, 140–41
Gorbachev, Mikhail, 125
Gray, Colin, 28, 73, 74, 75
Grisez, Germain, 134, 187, 188, 203, 204, 206–8, 210, 211, 217
Gumbleton, Thomas, 124

Hard-target kill capability, 19, 75
Hard targets, 113
Häring, Bernard, 190, 206
Harvard Nuclear Study Group, 4
Hauerwas, Stanley, 65–68, 70, 164, 167, 171
Hehir, Bryan, 4, 123
Heidelberg Theses of 1959, 141, 145
Hessian Institute for Peace Research, 124
Hiroshima, 49, 166
Hoffman, Stanley, 3, 4, 72
Hollenbach, David, 37, 168, 201; just-war thesis and, 45–49
Human rights, 3, 61, 65, 67, 75, 128, 153–54, 204

ICBMs, 107
In Defense of Creation, 165–66
Innocents. *See* Noncombatants
Intelligence, improvements in, 137
Intention, 5, 14, 16, 17, 18, 21, 29, 35, 41, 45, 46, 48, 49, 64, 71, 81, 85, 86, 91, 96, 101, 111, 131
Intentio recta, 147
Intermediate Nuclear Forces (INF), 125,

126, 140, 145; debate over, 142, 144; negotiations over, 13
Intermediate Nuclear Forces (INF) Treaty, 125
International law, 97, 103

Johann, Robert, 190
John Paul II, 129, 133; nuclear deterrence and, 130
Johnson, James Turner, 1, 35, 37, 65, 161
John XXIII, 2
Jus ad bellum, 4, 45, 96, 97, 109, 110, 147
Jus ante et contra bellum, 4
Jus in bello, 4, 45, 96–98, 107, 109, 110, 112, 113, 129, 130, 131, 134, 146, 147
Justa causa, 147
Just and Unjust Wars, 17
Just cause, 14, 97, 98, 102, 109
Justice, 170; definition of, 153; distributive, 3; peace and, 169
"Justice, Peace and the Preservation of Creation," 145
Justification, 128
Just peace, doctrine of, 149–55
Just-war doctrine, 130, 148, 154, 155; definition of, 95–96
Just-war theory, 16, 63, 67, 71, 73, 85, 88, 98, 103, 110, 123, 126, 132, 134, 135, 138, 152, 163, 196; ethical problems of, 146–49
Just-war tradition, 1–3, 14, 18, 25, 35, 60–62, 64, 65, 70, 72, 75, 79, 80, 91, 95, 97–99, 102–4, 106–9, 112, 114–15, 146, 147, 149, 165, 174, 192, 197, 198, 200, 201, 208; criticism of, 40–49; pacifism and, 162–64, 166–73, 176, 177, 212

Kellogg-Briand Pact, 151
Kenny, Anthony, 29, 31; deterrence and, 15–17
King, Martin Luther, 165
Kingdom of God, 6, 67, 70, 174, 175; "already," 172, 176; "not yet," 173, 176. *See also* Reign of God; Second Coming
Kirchentag, 145

Komonchak, Joseph, 213
Krell, Gerd, 124
Krol, John Cardinal, testimony of, 83–84

Lammers, Stephen, 63–64
Langendörfer, Hans, 124
Lasers, moral defensibility of, 107
Last resort, 79, 96–98, 201
League of Nations Covenant, 97
Leo XIII, 223
Limitation, principles of, 14
Limited nuclear war, 18–20, 41, 42, 132;
    ethics and, 71–76
Living With Nuclear Weapons, 4

MacIntyre, Alasdair, 54, 55, 66–69
Mackie, J. L., 38
McKim, Robert, 37
McNamara, Robert, 15
Mara, Gerald, exceptionalist thesis and,
    52–55
Meehan, Francis X., 163, 174, 201
Mendes-France, Pierre, 89
Methodist bishops, 37, 166–67, 169, 171,
    172, 175–76; statement of, 165–66
Military force, role of, 151–52
Minuteman missiles, 74, 112
MIRVs, 74, 76
Morality, 89, 155, 185; differences in, 52;
    religion and, 69; violating, 51
Moral reason: crisis of, 59; deontological
    approaches to, 134
Mouw, Richard, 169
Murray, John Courtney, 1
Mutual assured destruction (MAD), 22,
    37, 64, 71–75, 83; objections to, 28
MX missiles, 74

National sovereignty, 4
NATO, 18, 84, 108, 132, 140, 144,
    145, 204
Nazi Germany, Protestant churches and,
    140, 141
Neutron warheads, 108
*New Call to Peacemaking of the Historic
    Peace Churches,* 164
New "dark ages," description of, 66–67
New Testament, 150

Niebuhr, H. Richard, 161, 189–99, 209,
    213, 217, 219–21
Niebuhr, Reinhold, 1, 89, 161
Nitze, Paul, 29
No-first-use policy, 13, 18, 23, 25,
    26, 121
Noncombatant immunity, 1, 14–16, 18,
    19, 21, 40, 45, 50, 54, 62–65, 67,
    68, 80, 100, 102, 107–10, 170, 192,
    197, 201
Noncombatants, 17, 22, 24, 26, 49, 63,
    64, 75, 84, 86, 96–98, 100, 101, 102,
    106, 107, 109–15, 130, 131, 133, 135,
    146, 186, 197, 202
Nonviolence, 165, 168, 174, 175. *See also*
    Pacifism
Novak, Michael, 86
*Nuclear Deterrence, Morality, and
    Realism,* 187
Nuclear Ethics, 1, 25
Nuclear Freeze, 30
Nuclear-free zones, 144
Nuclear pacifism, 15, 20, 21, 41, 45, 48,
    81, 82, 84, 85, 91, 103, 114, 124,
    144. *See also* Disarmament; Pacifism;
    Unilateralism
Nuclear strategy: ethics and, 14;
    World War II and, 139
Nuclear weapons: improvements in,
    109–14; moral assessment of, 128–29
Nuclear winter, 81, 103, 113
Nye, Joseph, 1, 4, 17, 30, 31; strategy of,
    25–27

Obliteration bombing. *See* Saturation
    bombing
O'Brien, William V., 14–15, 26, 65,
    73, 74, 123; MAD and, 37
Old Testament, 150
Out of Justice, Peace, 143

Pacem in Terris, 2
Pacifism, 55, 71, 121, 124, 149, 165, 174,
    175, 192, 196, 200, 201; alternative
    of, 65–70; deterrence and, 167; just-
    war tradition and, 162–64, 166–73,
    176, 177, 212. *See also* Disarmament;
    Nuclear pacifism

Pact of Paris, 97
Pastoral Constitution on the Church in the Modern World (Gaudium et Spes), 2, 195, 198, 200
Pastoral letter. See *The Challenge of Peace*
Patria, 55
Pax Christi, 124
Payne, Keith, 28
Peace: concept of, 148–51; justice and, 169
Peacemaking, Christian, 164, 167, 174, 177
"Peace of God," 148
"Peace Order Concept," 148
Pershing II missiles, 112, 125
Pius XII, 2, 194, 223
Plausibility, 211–13, 215, 222–24; case for, 216–17; constraints on, 209–10; definition of, 195–96; philosophical considerations of, 205–9
Polis, 54, 55
Post-Enlightenment philosophy, 54, 66
Potter, Ralph, 1
Pragmatic realism, 213
"The Preservation, Promotion and Renewal of Peace," 142
Prima facie duties, 98
Proportionality, 1, 6, 14, 16, 22, 27, 40, 41, 46, 62, 67, 73, 80, 88, 97, 107, 108, 110–12, 126, 128–32, 135–37, 146–47, 170, 192, 197, 201, 206
Protestant churches, 3; Nazi Germany and, 140, 141
Public authority, 5
Putnam, Hilary, 206, 209–12

The Quest for Peace, quotation from, 161

Radical Monotheism and Western Culture, 220
Ramsey, Paul, 1, 14–15, 21, 23, 24, 26, 70, 101, 110, 111, 167, 203
Rationalism, 212; post-Weberian, 54
Ratzinger, Cardinal, 183
Reagan, Ronald, 27, 28, 89, 104, 125
Reagan administration, 13, 125, 221
Reasoning, 189
Reformed Church, 143, 144

Reign of Christ, 170
Reign of God, 171. *See also* Kingdom of God; Second Coming
"The Relation of the Church to the War in Light of the Christian Faith," 193
Relativism, 205, 208–9
The Renunciation of the Spirit and Logic of Deterrence, 144–45
Response, 192, 213–14; fittingness of, 191
Responsibility, 190–91
The Responsible Self, 189, 191, 193, 195
Responsive-magisterial approach, 181, 182, 189, 196, 216–20, 223, 224
Retaliation, 80, 88, 99, 100
Right authority, 97
Right intention, 97
Risse, Heinz-Theo, 124
Risse-Kuppen, Thomas, 124
Ross, W. D., 207
Rule of law, 149
Russett, Bruce, 123
Russian Orthodox Church, 145

St. Benedict, 67, 69
Saturation bombing, 1, 62, 63, 65, 95
Schell, Jonathan, 113, 135
Schmidt, Darrell, 168
Schmidt, Hans-Joachim, 124
Schmidt, Helmut, 126
Scowcroft commission, 74
Second Coming, 142. *See also* King of God; Reign of God
Second-strike counterforce, 28, 40, 41, 43, 44, 114
Second Vatican Council, 2, 18, 60, 127, 131, 192, 195, 199, 200
Self-defense, 26, 50
Self-preservation, 154–55
Shalom, 165, 171, 176; definition of, 164
Sider, Ronald, 164
Social contract theory, 67–68, 70
Social Principles, 167–68
Social solidarity, 191, 194–95
The Social Sources of Denominationalism, 221
Society of Christian Ethics, 164
Soft targets, 113
Sojourner Community, 164

Soviet Union, 104, 112, 132, 139, 175; deterring, 22
Status confessionis, 141, 143–45. *See also* Confessing Church
Stein, Walter, 18, 29, 31; deterrence and, 15–17
Strategic Defense Initiative (SDI), 5, 27, 28, 35, 95, 96, 103, 112, 115; description of, 104–8; moral defensibility of, 107
Strategy, ethics and, 28–31
Success thesis, 36–39, 55
Supreme emergency, 5, 6, 35, 53, 55, 62, 63, 67, 68, 135, 220; criticism of, 49–52; definition of, 17

Targeting policy, 26, 102, 114, 136. *See also* Countercity targeting
Teleology, 69–70, 128, 129, 133, 190, 192, 196, 197, 206
Test ban treaty, 19
Thatcher, Margaret, 89
Thomas Aquinas, 61, 67, 85, 96, 186
Threat, 14, 21, 35, 47, 48, 50, 52, 60, 65, 71, 74, 79, 80, 90, 91, 96, 101, 102, 111. *See also* Deterrence
Tradition, reformulating, 6
Tranquillitas Ordinis, 168
Troeltsch, Ernst, 161

Unilateralism, 154, 155, 188, 197, 203, 211, 217. *See also* Disarmament; Nuclear Pacifism
United Nations Charter, 97

U.S. Catholic Conference, 123
Utilitarianism, 67, 68, 70, 128, 129, 134, 135, 206; rejection of, 3
Vanderpol, Albert, 96
von Weizacker, Carl Friedrich, 145

Walzer, Michael, 5, 6, 21, 53, 54, 61–65, 68, 71–73, 134, 135, 220; deterrence and, 17–18; supreme emergency and, 49–52
War-fighting strategies, 19, 75, 99, 106–8, 111, 112
Warsaw Pact, 60, 132
Wasserstrom, Richard, 36, 39, 48
Weigel, George, 168, 169, 172
Weinberger, Caspar, 36, 38
White, Morton, 206, 207, 208
Wieseltier, Leon, deterrence and, 37
Wohlstetter, Albert, 2, 23, 24, 26, 29, 65, 73–75; strategy of, 20–22
Woodstock Theological Center, conference at, 123, 124
World Council of Churches, assembly of, 145
World Court, 97
World Health Organization, 150, 151
World order, 3
World War I, 146
World War II, 146; nuclear strategy and, 139

Yoder, John Howard, 65, 103, 164

Zuckerman, Solly, 37